P9-BYY-285

the Abs Diet
Ultimate Nutrition Handbook

the Abs Diet
Ultimate Nutrition Handbook

Your Reference Guide to Thousands of Foods, and How Each One Shapes Your Body

DAVID ZINCZENKO

Editor-in-Chief of **Men'sHealth.**

WITH TED SPIKER

RODALE

Notice

This book is intended as a reference volume only, not as a medical manual. The information given here is designed to help you make informed decisions about your health. It is not intended as a substitute for any treatment that may have been prescribed by your doctor. If you suspect that you have a medical problem, we urge you to seek competent medical help.

Mention of specific companies, organizations, or authorities in this book does not imply endorsement by the author or publisher, nor does mention of specific companies, organizations, or authorities imply that they endorse this book, its author, or the publisher.

Internet addresses and telephone numbers given in this book were accurate at the time it went to press.

Some portions of this book have appeared previously in *Men's Health* magazine.

© 2007 by Rodale Inc.

All rights reserved. No part of this publication may be reproduced or transmitted in any form or by any means, electronic or mechanical, including photocopying, recording, or any other information storage and retrieval system, without the written permission of the publisher.

Rodale books may be purchased for business or promotional use or for special sales. For information, please write to:

Special Markets Department,
Rodale Inc., 733 Third Avenue, New York, NY 10017

The Abs Diet and *Men's Health* are registered trademarks of Rodale Inc.

Printed in the United States of America

Rodale Inc. makes every effort to use acid-free ∞, recycled paper ♻.

Photographs pages 142–44, 146–47, 150, 152–57: © Beth Bischoff
Page 145: Mitch Mandel/Rodale Images
Pages 149 and 151: John P. Hamel/Rodale Images

Book design by Chris Rhoads

Library of Congress Cataloging-in-Publication Data

Zinczenko, David.
    The abs diet ultimate nutrition handbook : your reference guide to thousands of foods, and how each one shapes your body / David Zinczenko ; with Ted Spiker.
        p.   cm.
    Includes index.
    ISBN-13 978–1–59486–757–6   hardcover
    ISBN-10 1–59486–757–7   hardcover
    1. Nutrition—Handbooks, manuals, etc.   2. Weight loss—Handbooks, manuals, etc.   3. Exercise—Handbooks, manuals, etc.   I. Spiker, Ted.   II. Title.
    RA784.Z56   2007
    613.2—dc22   2007019096

Distributed to the trade by Holtzbrinck Publishers

2   4   6   8   10   9   7   5   3   1   hardcover

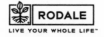

We inspire and enable people to improve their lives and the world around them

For more of our products visit **rodalestore.com** or call 800-848-4735

www.theAbsDiet.com

Contents

Introduction

EVERYWHERE YOU TURN, you have to make a decision. Take the call or send it to voice mail? Delete the ex's e-mail or cyber-flirt in a reply? Send the kids to public or private? The black shoes or brown? Grande or venti? 1-866-IDOLS-07 or 1-866-IDOLS-08? With all the decisions you make every day, I know that you've got a lot on your plate.

Your metaphorical full plate, unfortunately, also leads to a literal one. With all of life's stresses, responsibilities, and pressures, you probably don't take even a second to make one of the most crucial decisions of your life: what to eat. We've become a society that's busier than ever—and, in turn, fatter than ever. The link is clear: The busier you are, the less likely you are to consider what you're about to shovel in your mouth and the more likely it is to end up padding your stomach.

Smart eating comes down to smart decision making. It's not about elaborate recipes or prepackaged plans or revolving every meal around sausage and cheese, and it's not about depriving yourself of food so that you slip into a state of hallucinatory hunger. It's about making good, simple decisions meal to meal, bite to bite. Of course, the only way you can make smart decisions is by being armed with the right information about what foods are destined to make you lean and which ones are destined to make your belly look like a hot-air balloon.

That's exactly what *The Abs Diet Ultimate Nutrition Handbook* is for—to give you the information you need to make smart decisions, whether you eat in or out, in your car, at your desk, with your family, by yourself, on the go, or over the sink. No matter what your lifestyle, the Abs Diet is a simple, effective, and doable eating-and-exercise plan that will transform your body and give you the flat stomach and strong body you want. How? By giving you the nutritional principles you can use every time you want to add something else to your plate.

The Abs Diet: The Ultimate Nutrition and Exercise Plan

THE REASON I'm so passionate about the Abs Diet is because I know it works. I've heard from the thousands of men and women who have embraced the Abs Diet principles and changed their bodies and lives forever. Now, as the sixth book in the Abs Diet series, *The Abs Diet Ultimate Nutrition Handbook* gives you even more nutrition secrets—information and inspiration that you can use every time you eat. I know you'll find this book to be helpful, considering that a University of California, Berkeley, study found that nearly a third of the average person's diet is pure junk that provides no nutritive value, just calories. You'll be able to use this book's secrets along with the Abs Diet principles to get away from your junkyard diet and pack your meals with nutrient-rich Powerfoods that help burn more fat, build muscle, and change your body.

While this book centers around eating, nutrition, and food, I think it's worth mentioning here that one reason the Abs Diet is so effective is that it combines both sound eating and exercise plans—something lacking in so many weight-loss programs. A Brazilian study found that diet controls about 75 percent of weight loss—meaning that a smart eating plan is certainly the foundation for the most effective program, but it's not the only thing to focus on if you want results. Consider this research: A Wake Forest University study showed that people who diet and exercise shrink their abdominal fat cells twice as much as those who diet only—even when they lose the same amount of total weight. When scientists analyzed the body-fat distribution of study participants who had dropped an average of 22 pounds, they found that those who included exercise in their weight-loss programs were able to specifically target belly fat. The researchers theorize that because abdominal fat cells may have different amounts of metabolic enzymes than other parts of the body, they may be more responsive to exercise. I've included an abridged version of the Abs Diet Workout on page 139, and I've also added new workouts for those of you already familiar with the exercise programs.

If you're new to the Abs Diet, you'll embrace its simplicity and effectiveness—and, most of all, how darn satisfying it is. These are the main nutrition principles of the Abs Diet.

Eat six meals a day. The Abs Diet isn't simply about revealing your abdominal armor. To lose weight and change your shape, you've got to raise your metabolic rate to burn more calories—even when you're not exercising. One of the main ways to keep your metabolism stoked is by constantly feeding (we're not talking about buffet troughs, mind you). If you eat six times a day—in the form of three meals and three snacks—you'll avoid the daily metabolic highs and lows that make you more likely to overeat. Study after study supports the effectiveness of eating frequent, high-nutrient meals. One study in the *American Journal of Epidemiology*, for instance, found that people who ate four or more meals a day had half the risk of becoming overweight, compared with those who ate three or fewer times daily. Ideally, at each meal, you'll have a good mix of protein, good-for-you carbohydrates, and healthy fat to stave off hunger and keep you satisfied throughout the entire day. Which leads to the next Abs Diet principle . . .

Base your meals on the 12 Powerfoods. You'll meet them up close in a few pages, but the foundation of the Abs Diet is this: Eat most of your foods from these 12 groups of Powerfoods—which give you literally hundreds of choices—and you'll take control over your body, rather

than having your body control you. Learn the 12, love the
12, live by the 12.

Almonds and other nuts
Beans and legumes
Spinach and other green vegetables

Dairy (fat-free or low-fat milk, yogurt, and cheese)
Instant oatmeal (unsweetened, unflavored)
Eggs
Turkey and other lean meats

Peanut butter
Olive oil
Whole-grain breads and cereals
Extra-protein (whey) powder
Raspberries and other berries
12!

Drink smoothies. Here's a problem I have with most
diets: They leave your stomach growling and howling like
category 5 winds. I've said it before, but if there's one thing
that's the clear path to successful weight loss, it's the same
thing that keeps lovers and Rolling Stones fans happy: satisfaction. Your stomach has to be satisfied by being filled (yet
not overstuffed). Your body has to be satisfied it's getting
the right nutrients, and your tongue has to be satisfied
with the variety of tastes it's experiencing. If you find yourself unsatisfied in the form of such things as extreme hunger
or extreme blandness, then there's only one possible outcome,
and it's not pretty: You'll find yourself diving nose-first into
an entire cheesecake.

That's why I love smoothies so much: Integrate them
as regular meals or snacks, and you'll more than fill your
quota of satisfaction. Now, I'm talking about homemade
ones, not necessarily store-bought ones, which can be
pumped full of sugar and other fattening ingredients. Just
dump several healthful ingredients (milk, yogurt, chocolate
whey powder, berries, for instance) into a blender and you

have yourself a filling meal that's just as sweet as any bad-for-you belt-buster.

Stop counting. Calories are like votes—they're all important, but I wouldn't want to be in charge of counting every single one. Going back to the fact that most of us are busier than a beer vendor at a football game, I know you don't have time to measure, weigh, and count everything you put in your mouth. That's why I've designed the Abs Diet so you don't have to measure, weigh, or count. Just be aware of the Powerfoods and eat them regularly, and the calories will essentially count themselves. How? You'll eat often enough and with enough nutritional diversity that you'll stay full and satisfied all day long—rather than experiencing the blood-sugar surges that can cause you to annihilate everything in your pantry.

Don't waste calories on drinks. Here's the thing about drinks: You can down most of them so fast that it's like funneling excess calories and sugar into your bloodstream to eventually be stored as fat. Think of most drinks as bad TV—time spent with them will likely be a waste. With a few exceptions—like low-fat milk, vegetable juice, and occasional 100 percent fruit juices—you should avoid caloric drinks. While a moderate amount of alcohol a day (one to two drinks) has been shown to have a protective

WHAT HAVE YOU GOT TO LOSE?

In weight-loss circles, we get pounded with messages the way paparazzi get pounded with middle fingers. One of the biggest messages: Take it slow, and be realistic about how much you want to weigh. While it's clear that you can't shed fat instantly, it doesn't hurt to be aggressive about your weight-loss and body-changing goals. University of Minnesota researchers found that having high expectations may help you lose more weight. They found that those who tried to lose an average of 16 percent of their body weight—instead of the commonly recommended 5 to 10 percent—did indeed drop more pounds than their conservative counterparts.

effect on the heart, I want you to limit your alcoholic drinks to a few (or none) a week, and drop the sodas and energy drinks. I'm not much for counting calories per se, but you do need to think about where you want to spend them; if a drink doesn't qualify as a Powerfood (milk and vegetable juices do), then opt for something else. And don't forget about the ultimate no-calorie beverage: plain old water. You'll be amazed at what happens to your hunger if you sub in two glasses of water before every meal.

Cheat. You heard me right: Cheat when you eat. Once a week, indulge in your favorite meal or dessert or appetizer or whatever it is that's been taunting you like a trash-talking baller. Indulge your cravings now and then, and you'll be much more likely to stick to your Powerfoods the rest of the time. Time and time again, I hear from folks who say they love having the cheat-meal option, yet once they get to that meal, they're so happy with their Powerfoods that they rarely feel the need to gorge on triple cheeseburgers.

The Abs Diet: The Foundation for Success

HOW DO YOU MAKE all this work? Easy. Just spend a little bit of time each day planning what you're going to eat and when. That small amount of preparation will take out the indulgent nature of failed diets—you eat *anything* because you've thought of *nothing*. According to a University of Washington study, 64 percent of men spend little or no time preparing their meals (coincidence that 64 percent are overweight?). Worse, the inexpensive foods we tend to reach for are the ones with fat, sugar, and calories.

I'm convinced that one of the major behavioral shifts you can make to change your body is to change your thinking. I'm not asking you to spend hours preparing recipes, and I'm not asking you to wield cooking utensils like a baton twirler. I'm just asking that you take 10 minutes a day to think about what you're going to eat and prepare the easy-to-make things in advance—bag up your daily snacks, mix up a smoothie for tomorrow's breakfast. A couple of minutes a day can save you a couple of dozen pounds a year.

I know the Abs Diet works, not only because of all of the success stories from those who've crossed over to this lifestyle, but also because the Abs Diet principles, recommendations, and Powerfoods are backed by science that shows this type of program will help you lose weight. Consider one study in which researchers at the Centers for

WHAT'S IN YOUR BELLY FAT?

Six-pack abs aren't just about vanity; they're the sign of a healthy body. That's because the fat that settles around your belly secretes substances known as adipokines, which raise your risk of disease. In fact, the larger your midsection grows, the more dangerous it becomes. If the image of a bulbous belly isn't enough to make your stomach turn, take a close look at what your belly fat is producing.

▶ **Resistin:** a hormone that leads to high blood sugar, an independent risk factor for diabetes and heart disease

▶ **Plasminogen activator inhibitor:** a substance that contributes to the formation of blood clots, which can cause heart attacks and strokes

▶ **Interleukin-6:** a chemical that causes arterial inflammation, which can trigger pieces of plaque to break off arterial walls and block the flow of blood to the heart

▶ **Angiotensin:** a compound that raises blood pressure

▶ **Adiponectin:** an anti-inflammatory compound that helps counteract the effects of interleukin-6. Unfortunately, as fat cells grow larger, the amount of adiponectin they secrete usually decreases.

Disease Control and Prevention surveyed nearly 600 successful dieters and found that:

▶ 71 percent ate more fruits and vegetables (part of the Abs Diet!)

▶ 36 percent planned meals (part of the Abs Diet!)

▶ 19 percent lifted weights (part of the Abs Diet!)

But that's just the beginning. As editor-in-chief of *Men's Health* magazine, I'm tuned in to all the latest nutritional research, and that's why I've put together *The Abs Diet Ultimate Nutrition Handbook*—to give you information you can use at every meal, as well as some of the latest and greatest secrets about food and nutrition. Remember, every decision you make about what you put on your plate directly influences whether or not it will end up on your stomach.

And that begs the question about whether you're ready to make the biggest decision of all: Are you destined to a life of tight pants, or are you ready to buy some new ones?

Chapter I

THE POWER 12
The Powerfoods That Will Shrink Your Waist and Change Your Body—Forever

POWER COMES FROM ALL KINDS of sources. For a car, it's gasoline. For your new plasma TV, it's electricity. For bedroom toys, it's a pair of double-A Duracells. For you? It's food. Food is your fuel, your electricity, your nutritional battery pack. Food not only gives you the ability and energy to move, live, work, and play, but it also gives you the power to change your body—for better or worse.

You already know full well what the bad ingredients (like sugar, saturated fat, and high-fructose corn syrup) can do. On the flip side, food can flatten a bulging middle if you douse your body with good-for-you ingredients like protein, whole-grain carbohydrates, unsaturated fats, fruits, vegetables, and fiber.

Easy in theory but tougher in practice, when we're so often tempted by restaurant menus, misleading marketing on food packages, and carnival foods. That's why I created the Abs Diet Power 12, an easy-to-remember, easier-to-implement eating plan that gives you the ability to eat properly at home, restaurants, business dinners, parties, ballparks . . . anywhere. Remember this simple formula, base your meals around these foods, and you'll power yourself with the fuel that'll steer your body in any direction you want.

Almonds and other nuts
Beans and legumes
Spinach and other green vegetables

Dairy (fat-free or low-fat)
Instant oatmeal (unsweetened, unflavored)
Eggs
Turkey and other lean meats

Peanut butter
Olive oil
Whole-grain breads and cereals
Extra-protein (whey) powder
Raspberries and other berries
12!

Almonds and Other Nuts

FOR A LONG TIME, nuts were the Robert Downey Jr. of the supermarket—they got a lot of bad press, though there was an awful lot to like about them. They had the rap of having too many calories and too much fat and destroying too many intestinal tracts. But nuts are rich in monounsaturated fats—meaning that they help increase the amount of good cholesterol in your body to help clear your arteries. They're also high in protein, which helps build muscle and keeps you satiated throughout the day. That's why I consider them the ultimate snack. Include a couple of handfuls throughout the day (don't overload, because they are indeed high in calories); aim for up to 70 almonds a day (15 to 20 as a snack). That's the number that people in one study ate daily for 6 months, in conjunction with a reduced-calorie diet, to drop 18 percent of their body weight. Go for whole almonds, dry-roasted or in their unsalted, raw state.

INCLUDES:

Almonds and other nuts
Pumpkin and sunflower seeds
Avocados (fruit with a mild, nutlike flavor)

DOESN'T INCLUDE:

Salted or smoked nuts

Beans and Legumes

GROWING UP, we knew beans as side dishes at barbecues. Now that we're older, we know a bean's exact place in the kitchen: everywhere. Beans are such a powerful food— high in protein and satiating fiber—that they're one of the staples that will help you build muscle, burn fat, and refrain from feasting on Ding Dongs. Beans are your pantry's ultimate handyman—because of their versatility. You can serve them as side dishes or dump them in chili, burritos, soups, and salads.

INCLUDES:

Beans

Lentils

Peas

Chickpeas

Edamame

Hummus

DOESN'T INCLUDE:

Baked beans (high in sugar)

Refried beans (many are high in saturated fat)

Spinach and Other Green Vegetables

LET'S FACE IT: Vegetables have about as much sex appeal as a laser printer. But the fact is that the produce aisle is exactly where you'll find many of the disease-fighting, belt-shortening foods you should include in your diet. While some vegetables are packed with fiber (like broccoli), others are also rich in vitamins (like spinach). More subtly, they help satisfy the common crunch craving, keeping you away from button-popping chips, crackers, and cookies. My suggestion: Get a week's worth of crunchy vegetables, cut them up, and store them in the fridge. Reach there for them at night, or pack some for lunch.

INCLUDES:

Cruciferous vegetables (like broccoli and cauliflower)
Green, yellow, orange, and red vegetables

DOESN'T INCLUDE:

Vegetables fried or drenched in butter or cheese

Dairy

FOR ALL THE GOOD that dairy products do, we ought to expand milk mustaches to full-on beards. More and more evidence suggests that calcium and dairy products—long recognized as essential to bone health—are also crucial for weight loss. One study found that the daily consumption of three or more servings of dairy foods seems to target belly fat. In fact, people with the highest intakes had the leanest midsections—by an average of nearly 2 inches. The calcium that accompanies dairy foods may block fat absorption and make fat less likely to be stored in the abdominal region, according to researchers. Another bonus: A Swedish study found that eating dairy foods may cut the risk of heart attack by up to 38 percent. Finally, pouring on the milk helps because liquid takes up a lot of space in your stomach and helps you avoid all-out brownie binges.

INCLUDES:

Fat-free or low-fat milk, yogurt, cheese, and cottage cheese

DOESN'T INCLUDE:

Whole milk and frozen yogurt

Instant Oatmeal

ONE OF THE CHANGES you'll make with the Abs Diet involves what you do with your spoon. Out: ice cream, pudding, and Froot Loops. In: oatmeal and high-bran cereal. When Harvard researchers analyzed diets of more than 27,000 men over 8 years, they found that guys who ate one serving of whole-grain foods daily weighed 2.5 pounds less than those who ate only refined grains. Oatmeal contains soluble fiber, so it stays in your stomach for a long time, attracting fluid. And when there's no room for other food, there's no desire for it. Oatmeal—especially when you cook it with low-fat milk and top it off with berries—is one of the fastest, best, and tastiest ways to add fiber to your diet, and a daily bowl of it may keep off the pounds.

INCLUDES:

Unsweetened and unflavored oatmeal
High-fiber cereals

DOESN'T INCLUDE:

Cereals with added sugar or high-fructose corn syrup

Eggs

YOU WASTED PLENTY OF THEM on Old Man Miller's house on Mischief Night, but no more. Once thought of as a no-no food because of a link to cholesterol, eggs have shed the reputation of being a nutritional nightmare. Actually, they're a great source of protein, and having them for breakfast sets you up for a perfect day of eating. Saint Louis University researchers found that people who eat eggs for breakfast consume fewer calories the rest of the day than those who skip eggs. In the study, people were given one of two breakfasts: two scrambled eggs, two slices of toast, and a tablespoon of reduced-calorie fruit spread; or a bagel, 2 tablespoons of cream cheese, and 3 ounces of nonfat yogurt. Even though the breakfasts were equal in calories, the egg eaters ate 264 fewer calories by the end of the day. Here's a trick: Nuke a whisked egg in a coffee mug. When it's cooked (in less than a minute), it'll fit perfectly on a whole-grain English muffin.

INCLUDES:

Eggs

DOESN'T INCLUDE:

Omelets made with high-fat cheese and even higher-fat bacon

Turkey and Other Lean Meats

MEAT MAY BE A NICKNAME for a softball player, bouncer, or muscular dunce, but it also refers to one of the pillars of the Power 12. Turkey and other lean meats provide the best sources of protein, allowing you to build the all-important muscle that will help you burn calories and fat. They'll satisfy you and keep you lean: Scientists at McMaster University in Hamilton, Ontario, found that eating more protein may reduce the fat around your midsection. People who ate 20 more grams of protein every day than the group average had 6 percent lower waist-to-hip ratios. Most people in the study made small adjustments, such as replacing ¾ cup of rice with half a chicken breast. I recommend that you work lean meats into all of your meals—plus a snack. Try a slice of Canadian bacon with eggs in the morning, grilled chicken on a lunchtime salad, and a piece of fish or lean meat for dinner. Snack on a slice or two of deli turkey or a small can of tuna and a glass of low-fat milk.

INCLUDES:

Lean steak, fish, turkey, and chicken
Shellfish
Canadian bacon

DOESN'T INCLUDE:

Sausage
Bacon
Fatty cuts of steak (like rib eye and T-bone)

Peanut Butter
(All-Natural, Sugar Free)

PARTLY THANKS TO a certain Reese's product, peanut butter has—for as long as I can remember—been portrayed as being as evil as an Anthony Hopkins character. While it's true that PB has a lot of calories and fat, what's more important is that it contains healthy fat to help keep you full and your arteries clean. One reason I especially like PB: It satisfies those guilty tastebuds of yours—the ones that crave food that *feels* bad for you. In fact, you should be integrating PB into your meals—just avoid the high-sugar versions, and don't bathe in the stuff. I like dropping a teaspoon or two into a blender when I'm making smoothies. I also recommend the ultimate PB&J: all-natural PB and berries on whole-grain bread.

INCLUDES:

All-natural, sugar-free peanut, almond, and cashew butters

DOESN'T INCLUDE:

Mass-produced sugary, trans-fatty peanut butter

Olive Oil

FOR A LONG TIME, Americans embraced low-fat diets as enthusiastically as they've embraced reality TV, equating a low-fat diet with a low-fat body. But nutritional researchers quickly realized that people were much more successful with weight loss and weight control when they included healthy fats in their diets. Healthy fats like olive oil control cravings and keep dieters from eating lots of calories later in the day (they offer artery-clearing benefits, too). While I don't recommend drinking the stuff by the glass, do use olive oil in salad dressings, as a vegetable dip, and for cooking lean meats.

INCLUDES:

Olive, canola, peanut, and sesame oils

DOESN'T INCLUDE:

Vegetable and hydrogenated vegetable oils
Trans fatty acids
Margarine

Whole-Grain Breads and Cereals

THOSE IN-THE-BASKET BREADS served at restaurants equal instant blubber. That's because breads, bagels, and many bakery products are made with refined flour—that is, flour that's stripped of all the good and healthy parts of a grain. But that doesn't mean that all breads and cereals are naughtier than certain beauty pageant title-holders. Whole-grain breads and cereals contain the good parts, providing fiber and many disease-fighting nutrients. Plus, whole grains serve as important heart protectors. The more whole grains you eat, the less likely you are to develop arterial inflammation. In a Centers for Disease Control and Prevention study of more than 13,000 people, those who ate nine servings of whole grains a day were 30 percent less likely to have high levels of inflammation than those who consumed three or fewer servings. One caution: A lot of marketing lingo is misleading. The only way to ensure that you're getting all good stuff and no refined stuff is to make sure your labels say "100 percent" whole wheat or whole grain.

INCLUDES:

100 percent whole-grain or whole-wheat breads, cereals, and pastas
Brown rice

DOESN'T INCLUDE:

Processed carbohydrates like white breads, bagels, and doughnuts
Imposter products labeled only "wheat"

Extra-Protein (Whey) Powder

LITTLE MISS MUFFETT knew what she was doing. To add more protein into your diet, add a scoop of whey protein powder to a smoothie or a glass of milk. Whey protein—a type of animal protein—contains the essential amino acids to build muscle and burn fat. It also serves as the basis for the perfect postworkout snack. Slurping down a whey-protein shake after exercising builds calorie-burning muscle. It helps prevent overeating, too. In a University of Toronto study, men who had a whey-protein shake 2 hours before hitting a buffet ate 200 fewer calories than those who had soy- or egg-based protein shakes. Blend together low-fat milk, ice, chocolate whey powder, a banana, and a few berries.

INCLUDES:

Whey powder
Ricotta cheese (contains whey protein)

DOESN'T INCLUDE:

Soy protein

Raspberries and Other Berries

I COULD SIT HERE and spout off about all of the health benefits of berries and other fruits—lots of fiber, lots of vitamins, lots of cancer-fighting nutrients—but I'm pretty sure you're well aware that fruit equals firepower. Studies even show that some fruits—like apples and grapefruit—contain a type of fiber called pectin, which has been shown to have satiating effects for up to 4 hours. Your job: Add them in wherever you can—to smoothies, in oatmeal and cereal, as part of snacks.

INCLUDES:

Berries and all fruits, especially apples and grapefruit

DOESN'T INCLUDE:

Jelly, which eliminates fiber and adds sugar

Chapter 2

YOUR METABOLIC ENGINE

How to Keep Your Body Burning Fat and Calories All Day Long

WHEN WE WERE KIDS, we were metabolic machines. We could eat hot dogs, mac-and-cheese, and enough junk to fill a landfill. But to counteract our less-than-stellar eating habits, we also spent hours outside riding bikes, playing ball, and frying ants with magnifying glasses (as opposed to hours on our duffs in front of Xboxes, like today's plump kids, but that's a whole other story). And then came college. We could drink all night, have diner food at 3:00 a.m., and still be in the best shapes of our lives. But as we got older, something happened to our metabolisms, our habits, and—in the process—our waistlines. We slowed down and we sprouted out.

Now the trick is to reverse that biological and behavioral trend by getting your metabolism to burn the way it used to. If you can do that—through eating the right foods and doing the right kind of exercise—then you'll be able to get your body into its best shape ever.

First, though, let's clear up exactly what metabolism is. While many people like to think it's as genetic as height, eye color, or a propensity of back hair, that's not the whole story.

Your metabolic rate—the rate at which your body burns energy—is broken down into three main elements.

Basal metabolic rate: Think about everything that happens in your body—the heart beats, blood moves, lungs expand, neurons fire, and your nether regions do somersaults at unexpected times. All that biological movement takes energy, and that's your basal metabolic rate—the energy expended when you're lying completely at rest, in the morning after sleep. This accounts for 60 to 70 percent of the total calories used up each day as your body works to do everything from making your lungs function to repairing damaged tissues. Your organ structure can't change (that is, not without a scalpel and a little anesthesia), but there is one thing that can: muscle mass. Muscle mass requires more energy to be maintained than fat, so you up your basal rate when you increase your muscle mass. More on this in a moment.

The thermic effect of food: You know that it's not actual cheeseburger hunks that get lodged in your arteries. Your body takes all the stuff you jam down your Powerfood hole and breaks it down into different things. It requires a lot of metabolic work to convert food into energy. Complex carbohydrates are broken down to simple sugars, fats to fatty acids, and protein to amino acids—all of which cells throughout your body use. This thermic effect is the cost of digesting, using, and storing food energy and accounts for 10 to 15 percent of your total daily metabolism.

Activity: You move, you lose. It's the classic form of metabolism that we all know—when you're active, you burn calories. You exercise, you burn calories. You shovel snow, you burn calories. You have sex, tap your foot, or walk up and down the lingerie racks, you lose calories. The funny thing is, this activity makes up only 15 to 30 percent of metabolism.

So where does that leave us? While we may not be able to control the rate at which we burn calories to keep our kidneys pumping, we can certainly take steps to increase metabolic rate in all three of the areas. Not coincidentally, many of the guidelines and principles of the Abs Diet are designed to do just that.

Metabolism Booster 1: Eat, Eat, Eat

IF THIS IS YOUR FIRST FORAY into the Abs Diet, then you may be surprised by the guideline of eating six times a day. Go to the bathroom six times a day? Sure. Check YouTube six times a day? Okay. Think about naked bodies six times a day? Of course. But eat? Is that for real?

Not only is it a heck of a lot more real than a stripper's chest, but it's vital. Eating often throughout the day is the key to revving your metabolism. When you don't eat often enough (typical "dieter" behavior), your body thinks it's in starvation mode, so it actually stores fat (for the famine it believes is coming) and inhibits weight loss. If you space your meals and snacks about 3 hours apart, you'll increase your body's ability to burn (of course, those six meals can't be gargantuan portions of edible gunk). And no matter how many times you've heard about the importance of starting your day with more than a shower and a shave, I'll repeat it: Not eating breakfast can reduce your metabolic rate by up to 10 percent. In a study of nearly 3,000 people, Harvard researchers found that those who ate breakfast every day were 44 percent less likely to be overweight (and 41 percent less likely to suffer from insulin resistance—a precursor to diabetes) than those who skipped it.

A bonus: South African researchers found that men who ate most frequently consumed 27 percent fewer calories than those who ate the least often. In fact, it's a double bonus: By eating often, you not only burn more throughout the day but you eat less, too.

Metabolism Booster 2: Increase Muscle— And Intensity

WHEN IT COMES TO LOSING weight through exercise, two things are crucial to revving your metabolism, and neither of them has to do with working out for hours upon hours on end.

The first factor is lifting weights (or using machines or bands or body weight) to increase lean muscle mass. Just to maintain themselves, your muscles burn at least 10 times more calories than fat does, even when you're at rest. So by adding a few pounds of muscle, you increase your body's daily energy expenditure. It's especially important as you get older; most men lose 1 percent of muscle mass a year after age 25, which is part of the reason we're more likely to gain weight as we age. You won't build muscle with traditional cardiovascular exercise, like running or cycling at

DON'T SLOW DOWN

Here are three things that could be causing your metabolism to downshift.

Drugs: Antidepressants can boost spirits but also cause metabolism to shift from gazelle-fast to slug-slow. If you gain weight on a common antidepressant (Paxil is one shown to slow metabolism), ask your doc about a switch to Wellbutrin, which can actually raise metabolism.

Stopping smoking: Of course it's a good thing that you stopped smoking—your lungs, your arteries, and your family all thank you. But the one seeming positive of nicotine is that it increases metabolism, most likely because your body is forced to expend extra energy trying to detoxify itself from the chemicals. When you stop smoking, your metabolism slows. You can counteract that effect with some of the metabolism boosters discussed in this chapter. And to directly deal with the adjustment to life without a smoke-smelling wardrobe, do this: Chew on a combination of Nicorette and Jolt gums. A study in the *American Journal of Clinical Nutrition* found that men who chewed nicotine gum (2 milligrams) spiked with 100 milligrams of caffeine experienced a 10 percent increase in metabolism.

Hormones: When your thyroid gland doesn't pump out enough hormone (that's called hypothyroidism), every metabolic process, including calorie burning, slows down. You'll need a blood test for a definitive diagnosis, but the condition can be treated with synthetic thyroid hormone.

one steady pace (though you will burn calories and increase your cardiovascular health).

That's not to discount all cardiovascular exercise, however. At least once a week, you should engage in a high-intensity interval workout—that is, doing a cardiovascular exercise but varying the intensity (1 minute high, followed by 1 minute low, and so on). That kind of cardio plan works similarly to weight training by burning loads of calories not only during exercise but afterward as well. As your body works to cool off and repair the microtrauma to your muscles, the after-burn alone can torch another 100 to 200 calories.

Also, there seems to be a benefit from combining these first two boosters. A University of Colorado study linked increased "energy flux" (the total number of calories your body processes in a day) to increased metabolism. Working out harder and eating more often—while keeping the over-all balance between the two the same—could also improve your ability to break down food.

Metabolism Booster 3: Pack In the Protein

YOU PROBABLY CAN GUESS how I feel about Atkins and other all-protein diets. I support them about as much as I support global warming. I simply don't like the way all-protein plans dismiss important and disease-fighting foods like fruits and whole-grain carbohydrates. But here's what I do support: protein, which is primarily found in lean meats like chicken, beef, and fish. Not only does protein help build muscle to work on your metabolism indirectly, it also has a direct effect. A British study found that people who ate a higher percentage of protein-based calories burned 71 more calories a day (that's 7.4 pounds a year) than those on low-protein diets. That's partly due to the thermic effect of food—it takes more energy for your body to break down pro-tein than other nutrients. As a bonus, protein is part of what satiates you, which is why I recommend you get a little protein with every meal and snack.

Metabolism Booster 4:
Get Going, Will Ya?

YOU CAN CERTAINLY BLAME a slowed metabolism on everything from loss of muscle to lack of meals, but don't forget this culprit: the fact that you spend most of your day sitting down, lying down, and moving at about the rate of an engineless train. As a kid, you had recess. In college, you walked everywhere and played pickup ball for 4 hours a night. Now you sit. You type. You e-mail and IM. And you spend about as much time with your butt on furniture as Ms. Spears does with hers in the tabloids. The worst part (besides the bedsores): According to a University of North Carolina Wilmington study, people gain an average of 17 pounds in just 8 months of working a sedentary job. When you stop moving so much, so do your metabolic motors. Taking direct aim at the third area of metabolism, you can go a long way toward improving your burn rate through not only exercise but everyday movement.

In addition to all of the traditional tactics to incorporate more moving time—using the stairs (instead of the elevator), using your mouth (instead of e-mail) to communicate with a co-worker—just making a conscious decision to do more tapping, twiddling, fidgeting, and walking will up your metabolic rate. For a look into the future, consider this: One writer I work with at *Men's Health* used a newfangled desk that allows workers to walk at a 1 mph rate—producing an unbelievable calorie burn, compared with sitting. The rate was slow enough that it didn't disrupt this guy's ability to write. Maybe someday we'll all be working in tricked-out, techno-equipped pseudogyms that will allow us to burn fat while we burn the midnight oil.

Metabolism Booster 5:
Make Every Bite Count

FACT IS, you'll make the most gains by hitting the major fat burners. But I also believe that, just like in sports and romance, the little things count more than you think. Here's one example: Catechins, the powerful antioxidants found in green tea, are known to increase metabolism. In a study published in the *American Journal of Clinical Nutrition*, participants who consumed 690 milligrams of catechins from green tea daily had significantly lower body mass indexes and smaller waist measurements than those in the control group. Another: Fish oil—like that in tuna and salmon—has been shown to boost metabolism by up to 400 calories a day. If you don't like fish, you can take a supplement (1 to 2 grams) to get similar benefits. Of course, tea and tuna alone aren't the answers, but if you can incorporate more into your meals, you'll be doing just what we're all after: burning more, storing less.

Chapter 3

99 NUTRITION SECRETS
Life-Changing Tips, Tricks, and Trivia about Food

BETWEEN THE INTERNET, 24-hour news networks, and kids who grew up memorizing the backs of baseball cards, the world is full of information experts. And that's great. If you want to know about the history of Greece, the career batting average of Mickey Mantle, or the number of pages in Charlie Sheen's affidavit history, there's an expert out there who can satisfy your curiosity. While I've got nothing against *Jeopardy* junkies or rotisserie baseball freaks, I also believe that the best facts are the ones that can be upgraded—upgraded into practical information that can help you change your life.

That's why I'm passing along these important facts about food; they can help you decide what goes in your mouth, so your body can decide what goes on your waist. Like I said in this book's introduction, weight loss—and maintaining your ideal body—has a lot to do with decision making. One or two or all of these 99 nutrition secrets will help you make the right decisions.

1

AFTER A WORKOUT, some people can't even think about chowing down on food, but others are hungrier than a *Survivor* contestant on day 39. Either way, your body needs fuel. A good choice: a 16-ounce glass of low-fat milk, following either weight training or a cardio workout. University of Connecticut researchers found that, like weight training, aerobic exercise breaks down muscle (but unlike pumping iron, it doesn't stimulate muscles to grow afterward). Consuming about 20 grams of high-quality protein (found in that glass of milk) ensures you'll get at least 6 grams of essential amino acids, the amount that's been shown to stop muscle breakdown after a workout.

2

CRAVING YOUR CHEAT DESSERT while shopping for your 32nd new cell-phone case? A Cinnabon Classic cinnamon roll (813 calories) has nearly 500 more calories than one from Au Bon Pain (350).

3

SUPERCHARGE YOUR RECIPES by adding some stealth Powerfoods in unexpected places. While making burgers for your next cookout, mix a cup or two of instant oatmeal with the meat. That'll bulk up the patties without bulking up the calorie content.

4

FISH IS PACKED with all-important protein and omega-3 fatty acids, but a little midday tuna offers even more rewards. Swedish researchers found that people who ate fish for lunch consumed 11 percent fewer calories at dinner than those who had beef, even though—get this—both lunches contained the same number of calories. Why? It seems that the protein in fish takes longer to digest than the protein in beef and chicken—which may help you feel fuller longer and cut your appetite later.

5

TRYING TO DECIDE between two fast-food burgers is like deciding which convicted felon you'd ask to house-sit while you're away on vacation. But even if you're making the move through the drive-thru for your cheat meal of the week, you can spare yourself some abdominal agony by making the right food choice. The McDonald's Quarter Pounder with Cheese has 160 fewer calories (510) than the Burger King Whopper (670 calories).

6

NO MATTER HOW HARD you try to navigate a restaurant menu, you'll likely be tripped up by hidden fat and calories, monster portions, and really bad foods masquerading as good ones. Sure, a small salad with oil and vinegar is reliably safe, but what's the fun in that? Your premeal strategy: Two hours before going out to eat, have a snack consisting of Powerfoods with healthy fat and fiber. Then order a salad or shrimp cocktail as soon as you sit down, so you're more likely to wave off the bread basket and save yourself some calories.

7

YOU KNOW HOW I FEEL about fiber: Big fan. Big, *big* fan. But you're not limited to cereals, fruits, and bean salads to reap the digestive rewards. A study from the University of Tromsø in Norway found that people who took daily fiber supplements for a month lost nearly twice as much weight as people who followed the same low-calorie diet but took placebo pills. The supplemental fiber—4 grams daily—did the same work as fiber from food: It made them feel full, so they ate less. The ingredient in those supplements: glucomannan, a type of soluble fiber sold as powder and caplets at vitamin stores.

8

LOTS OF DIETERS FAIL because of the second-to-last thing they do before going to bed: search the pantry for something crunchy or creamy—and then down it during their favorite late-night comedian's monologue. The way to combat the urge: Pick what you're going to have for your sixth meal of the day—and stick to it. Saint Louis University scientists found that nighttime bingers who ate a predetermined snack 90 minutes after dinner were able to shed 5 pounds in 2 months. Eating a fixed snack prevents overeating. You can have the same snack used in the study—¾ cup of fiber-rich cereal with ⅔ cup of low-fat milk.

9

OR FOR YOUR SIXTH MEAL of the day, munch on a handful of walnuts. One gram of walnuts contains 2.5 to 4.5 nanograms of a hormone called melatonin, which can help regulate sleep patterns.

10

SEARCHING FOR A SIDE DISH to replace your rice, bread, or refined-flour pasta? Cauliflower has 2.5 times more calcium than a potato.

11

SPEAKING OF SPUDS, people who consume the most potatoes— one serving 3 or 4 days a week—have a 14 percent greater risk of developing diabetes than those who eat the fewest servings.

12

A CERTAIN *SEINFELD* EPISODE elevated soup to unprecedented levels of popularity. And that's a good thing. Researchers at Pennsylvania State University found that snacking on soup can help speed weight loss. The study tracked people who followed reduced-calorie diets for a year. Those who ate one serving of soup twice a day lost 50 percent more weight than those who ate healthful but carbohydrate-heavy snacks, like baked chips or crackers. Now, cream-based soups don't count. Broth-based ones do.

13

CHEESE—AS IN cheese pizza, cheesecake, and cheeseburgers—deserves the bad press it gets because of all the saturated fat. But you don't have to eliminate all of it from your daily eating plan. In fact, go ahead and have one slice of hard or semihard cheese—Cheddar, Swiss, or provolone—for a snack. Cheese has 7 grams of protein per slice and contains no sugar, so your body stays in fat-burning mode.

14

IN BARS, convenience stores, and gyms, energy drinks have become the latest liquid rage. No bull: New Zealand scientists discovered that, despite the claim that they boost metabolism, many popular energy drinks are far worse for your gut than soda is. Why? They're often packed with sugar. The researchers found that an energy drink that contains 80 milligrams of caffeine and 24 grams of sugar—about the amount in a can of Red Bull—completely inhibited people's ability to burn fat. While caffeine does help speed metabolism, combining it with added sugar negates its short-term fat-burning benefits.

15

WE ALL TEND TO THINK that the power of oil and vinegar lies in the yellow stuff. But don't underestimate the red. A Swedish study found that people who consumed 2 tablespoons of vinegar with three slices of white bread had 23 percent lower blood-glucose levels than when they ate the bread alone (they also felt fuller). If you prefer to take your vinegar with salad, make your own salad dressing by mixing 2 tablespoons of olive oil with 2 tablespoons of vinegar.

16

THE ULTIMATE CONDIMENT: salsa. Low in calories, high in nutrients, goes with virtually everything.

17

WRITING DOWN WHAT YOU EAT can seem like as much of a waste of time as watching movie previews. But there's a reason the exercise works. Thinking about what you had for lunch keeps you from bingeing later on afternoon snacks. During a taste test, scientists asked people to rate three types of salted popcorn—and encouraged them to eat as much as they wanted. Those who were first asked to recall exactly what they had for lunch downed 30 percent less popcorn than those who weren't required to list their midday menu.

18

FRUITS ARE LIKE community volunteers; even if you don't like them personally, how can you complain about all the good they're doing? While it's true that all fruits deliver powerful nutrients, the USDA ranked the top 10 for disease-fighting antioxidants. The order:

Blueberries

Cranberries

Blackberries

Raspberries

Strawberries

Apples

Cherries

Black Plums

Avocados

Pears

19

IF YOU THINK EATING FISH is about as appealing as using your finger to hook it, consider the alternative of taking a fish-oil supplement. Australian scientists recently discovered that a combination of exercise and consumption of 6 grams of daily fish oil decreased body fat significantly more than exercise alone. Fish oil may stimulate enzymes that improve your body's ability to burn fat. More studies are needed to determine whether 6 grams is a safe amount, but you can get most of the benefit by taking 1 to 2 grams of fish oil a day.

20

TACO BELL JUNKIES, listen up. Arizona State University researchers found that eating ½ cup of pinto beans a day cuts LDL ("bad") cholesterol by 8 percent.

21

A STUDY FROM Texas Tech University and the Mayo Clinic suggests that people who have a daily alcoholic drink are 54 percent less likely to have a weight problem than those who don't imbibe. (Two drinks are also linked with less risk of overweight, but any more than that is trouble.)

22

REACH FOR PICKLES, not Pringles. Dill spears (1 calorie each) cover cravings for a salty, crunchy fix.

23

DOING THINGS BACKWARD may get you in trouble at work or in the bedroom but not necessarily in the kitchen. Consider having cereal for lunch a day or two a week. A Purdue University study shows that eating cereal in place of meals helps people lose weight, probably due to portion control with easy-to-prepare foods. Participants consumed an average of 640 fewer calories daily and lost roughly 4 pounds during the 2-week experiment. Stick to filling, high-fiber cereals like All-Bran or Fiber One (and low-fat milk).

24

A VENDING MACHINE is a dieter's kryptonite—it can make you very weak if you're exposed to it too long. If you must have a snack from a machine or a convenience store, your best bet is a PayDay. It's lower in sugar and calories than most candy bars, and because of the nuts, it has more fiber plus a high amount of the good unsaturated fat.

25

THOUGH IT USUALLY RIDES SHOTGUN in the citrus category, grapefruit packs some serious weight-loss power. Louisiana State University researchers found that people who ate half a grapefruit three times a day lost 4 pounds in 12 weeks— without deliberately altering any other part of their diet. They also lowered their blood pressure by 6 points, enough to reduce their risk of stroke by 40 percent. Researchers speculate that grapefruit's acidity may slow digestion, helping you stay full for longer periods of time.

26

YOU PROBABLY SAY THE WORDS "no time for breakfast" almost as often as you say, "Britney did what?" If that's the case, stash a workplace supply of Quaker Oatmeal Express, which comes in its own cup. Just add water and nuke for 30 seconds.

27

AT A PARTY, nibble on appetizers the way you'd sip a strong cocktail. Take it slow, and you'll avoid downing half a gallon of onion dip.

28

WHILE IT MAY BE RELAXING to have a fork in one hand and a remote in the other, a University of Massachusetts study found that people who watch TV during a meal consume 288 more calories than those who don't.

29

SPRINKLE 2 TEASPOONS of flaxseed over grilled chicken or fish for more texture and flavor.

30

A TRIP TO THE PRODUCE section can satisfy your desire for sweets. Really. Cornell University researchers found that fruit may satisfy a sweet tooth just as much as junk food does. When researchers examined the eating habits of more than 14,000 people, they found that those who ate the most baked goods also ate the most fruit. The connection: the sweetness. That means you may be able to calm your sugar cravings with a peach or a pear, rather than a sleeve of Thin Mints.

31

THE HEALTHIEST CUT OF BEEF: round. It comes from the rear end of the cow (pleasant visual, I know) and has the least amount of fat and the greatest amount of protein. Second best: loin.

32

GROUND TURKEY is a perfect substitute for ground beef in burgers, chili, and tacos—unless you're not careful. If you use dark-meat ground turkey, your burger will contain more fat, calories, and cholesterol than one made with 95 percent lean beef. Buy ground turkey made from breast meat only to benefit from this swap.

33

A MEDIUM TUB of movie theater popcorn has 1,120 calories. To burn it off, you'd have to climb the 1,665 stairs at the Eiffel Tower three times. Need a midflick crunch? Stash your own trail mix (made with nuts and dried fruit), and chomp on that.

34

FRUITS AND VEGETABLES are like skies and shoes—you can tell a lot about them by their color. Check this guide to health benefits according to hue.

> **Blues and purples** (blueberries, blackberries, plums, raisins, purple grapes, eggplant): improve memory and decrease cancer risk

> **Greens** (kiwifruit, honeydew, spinach, broccoli, romaine lettuce, Brussels sprouts, cabbage): protect bones, teeth, and eyesight

> **Whites** (bananas, pears, mushrooms, cauliflower, onions, garlic): lower LDL cholesterol and risk of heart disease

> **Reds** (watermelon, strawberries, raspberries, cranberries, cherries, tomatoes, red apples, radishes): help prevent Alzheimer's and improve bloodflow to the heart

> **Yellows and oranges** (oranges, grapefruit, peaches, cantaloupe, mangoes, squash, pineapple, carrots, corn): boost immune system and protect eyesight

35

ADDING FISH TO PASTA lightens up the noodles. When researchers in Britain topped pasta with tuna, they discovered that the glycemic index was cut in half. High-glycemic foods—such as pasta, bread, and potatoes—quickly raise blood-sugar levels, signaling the body to store fat. The protein in tuna helps slow the absorption of sugar into the bloodstream.

36

FINNISH RESEARCHERS found that refrigerating a cooked potato reduces its impact on blood sugar by 25 percent.

37

ADD A CUP OF RICOTTA to your fruit smoothie. The soft, mild cheese is made mostly of whey.

38

NUKING BROCCOLI may be the quickest way to destroy its health benefits. A Spanish study shows that microwaving destroys many of broccoli's disease-fighting nutrients—97 percent of its flavonoids, to be exact. Steaming retains all the nutrients.

39

AND YOU THOUGHT that a cap or razor was your only option for dealing with hair that disappears faster than David Blaine. Flax may actually halt receding hairlines. In a study, Taiwanese researchers put men who were losing their hair on 50 milligrams a day of lignans (phytonutrients found in flaxseed). Six months later, photos showed that hair loss had slowed in most of the men.

40

DROP A COUPLE OF CHUNKS of dark chocolate into your chili. Not only will it taste better (really), but it'll add flavonoids and polyphenols, nutrients that can lower your risk of heart disease and keep LDL cholesterol from oxidizing into an artery-damaging form.

41

YOU MAY APPRECIATE GRAPES for the fact that, when squished and squashed, they provide the base for a nice cocktail-party buzz. You might also eat a handful of them whole every day for added health benefits. Antioxidants in the skin of red grapes have been linked to lowering LDL cholesterol and preventing clogged arteries.

42

YES, SCARFING seafood helps you lose weight and look better on the beach. Even better, it helps you stay far away from the OR. In a study of more than 220,000 people, Northwestern University researchers were able to determine how much you can reduce the risk of heart disease by eating fish.

▶ One to three servings of fish per month: 11 percent reduction

▶ One per week: 15 percent

▶ Two to four per week: 23 percent

▶ Five or more per week: 38 percent

43

NEED ANOTHER REASON to eat more fish? University of Pittsburgh researchers found that omega-3 fatty acids may help relieve neck and back pain. Omega-3s seem to block inflammation and the accompanying pain.

44

MAKE CHILI CON CHICKEN: Grill a pound of chicken, slice it, and place it in a pan with 2½ cups of red chili beans, ⅓ cup of chicken stock, ¼ cup of barbecue sauce, and a can of diced tomatoes. Simmer for 10 minutes.

45

WASH DOWN YOUR AFTERNOON SNACK with a can of low-sodium V8—in men it cuts the risk of prostate cancer not only because of the lycopene in the tomatoes but also because of the high vegetable content.

46

IN THE DAIRY AISLE, opt for plain yogurt (top it yourself with fresh fruit) instead of the kind with fruit at the bottom, which contains more fructose (as in dangerous and fat-promoting high-fructose corn syrup).

47

THE ABS DIET BEER of choice: Amstel Light. It's 95 calories but doesn't taste like it.

48

THE ABS DIET WINE of choice: Pinot Noir. It supplies more disease-fighting antioxidants than any other alcoholic beverage.

49

WHILE THE ABS DIET discriminates against a few nutritional villains—saturated fat, trans fat, sugar, and high-fructose corn syrup—it's also a good idea to keep your carbohydrate intake under control. And, of course, you want to make sure the carbs you eat are the whole-grain variety. Some evidence for tipping your scale in favor of protein over carbs: University of Florida researchers found that dieters who eat less than 100 grams of carbohydrates daily lose an average of 4 pounds more fat a month than those whose carb intake is higher. The discovery was made when researchers analyzed 87 weight-loss studies comparing a variety of carbohydrate intakes, varying from 1 percent to 75 percent of the total calories consumed.

50

IF YOU'RE FOLLOWING the Abs Diet principles, then your blender is in the on position almost as much as your cell phone. And that's good. If you want to add a little more variety to your motorized meals, try this cold cucumber soup for a cool change of taste. Peel and chop an English cucumber—the long, skinny, seedless kind that usually comes wrapped in plastic—then dump it in a blender with 1 chopped shallot, ½ cup low-fat plain yogurt, 1 teaspoon extra-virgin olive oil, ¼ teaspoon dried dillweed, and a pinch each of salt and pepper. Blend until smooth, adding more yogurt, 1 tablespoon at a time, if needed to reach your desired consistency.

51

JARRED GARLIC SAVES TIME in the peel-and-chop process, but the precut stuff lacks many of the essential oils that impart the intense flavor. For the full garlicky effect, try mincing it yourself. Here's how: Lay a clove (still in its papery skin) on a cutting board. Place the blade of a heavy knife flat on top and whack it with your fist to flatten the clove. Peel off the skin and slice the clove lengthwise into thin planks. Rotate the slices 90 degrees and repeat for a fine mince and full garlic flavor.

52

SNACK ON THIS: 1 cup of 2 percent cottage cheese with ¾ cup of berries.

53

THE AVERAGE FREEZER packs everything from year-old meat to in-case-friends-stop-by beer mugs. Yours? Stock it with a make-your-own Powerfood dessert. Cut a slit in the foil cover of a 4-ounce container of low-fat flavored yogurt, then insert a wooden Popsicle stick. Freeze overnight. When you're craving sweets that'll last longer than a bite-size piece of chocolate, just run the carton briefly under hot water, peel back the foil, and pop out the frozen yogurt.

54

IF YOU LIKE VEGETABLES about as much as Simon Cowell likes karaoke, then you've got to find sneaky ways to integrate disease-busting veggies into your diet. Buy a fine grater disk for your food processor so you can mince them into microscopic bits that can then be hidden in ground beef or spaghetti sauce. Try this: Grate 2 cups (total) of onions, garlic, carrots, beets, spinach, and zucchini, then sauté in olive oil. Add 4 cups of marinara sauce and simmer.

55

A GOOD BREAKFAST won't just keep you from animalistic eating at the corner buffet; it'll also help you burn more calories during a workout. British scientists found that people who have a carbohydrate-rich, high-fiber breakfast before running burn twice as many calories. Why? Eating low-fiber, refined carbohydrates significantly raises the amount of insulin in your body, which limits your ability to use fat for fuel.

56

CHANCES ARE THAT WHEN you were growing up, spinach had the taste equivalent of soiled carpet. Still holding a grudge? Flavor your leafy greens with another Powerfood: turkey. Lightly coat the bottom of a large skillet with 2 teaspoons of olive oil and heat to medium-high. Add one crushed clove of garlic, three chopped slices of deli smoked turkey, and a pinch each of salt and black pepper. Stir until the garlic softens and the turkey begins to brown, then dump in an entire 10-ounce bag of baby spinach. It'll cook down to two servings. Turn frequently with tongs until the spinach is completely wilted (about 2 to 3 minutes) and see what you've been missing.

57

SOME PEOPLE SPIKE their glasses of water with lemon. Some do it with a tea bag. Some do it with that little bottle behind the bar. Here's something you can add to your water (you are getting eight 8-ounce glasses, right?): Fibersure. This new supplement from the makers of Metamucil packs 5 grams of fiber per teaspoon and dissolves flavorlessly into any liquid. Add it to water or your morning coffee, and you're well on your way to the 38 daily grams recommended by the USDA.

58

PROVOLONE HAS MORE calcium (211 milligrams per slice) and slightly fewer calories and less saturated fat than most other cheeses. Add a slice to your turkey whole-wheat wrap.

59

DON'T BE FOOLED by foods that sound healthier than they actually are. One of the most felonious offenders: granola, with saturated-fat levels higher than you'd find in a hamburger. If you're going to have it, buy the low-fat variety.

60

IT'S ABOUT TIME you caught some flax. Mix ¼ cup of flaxseed into your smoothie to add a whopping, stomach-satisfying 12 grams of fiber.

61

SUNDAYS ARE MADE for football, sleeping in, and *Desperate Housewives*. They're also made for prepping your refrigerator for a week of hassle-free eating. Cook 10 to 12 slices of turkey bacon, and store them in the fridge. During the next week, add a slice or two to a salad, a sandwich, or chili for extra protein, or have a few slices for a snack. You'll up your Abs Diet ante if you do the same with a couple of pounds of chicken breast.

62

I KNOW WHAT YOU'RE SAYING: There's only so much grilled chicken you can take before you start craving something more flavorful, like a pillow. But consider this: Chicken is like a naked body standing in a wardrobe full of clothes. To generate a little excitement, all you've got to do is change what it's wearing every once in a while. An idea for a sauce in which to marinate chicken for 30 minutes before grilling: ½ cup of balsamic vinegar, 2 tablespoons of Dijon mustard, 2 cloves of chopped garlic, and 2 tablespoons of chopped fresh rosemary.

63

OH, SO YOU NEED A FISH marinade, too? Mix 1 cup of olive oil, the juice of 1 lemon, 1 tablespoon of fresh thyme, and 2 cloves of chopped garlic.

64

OKAY, FINE; FOR BEEF: 1 cup of heavy red wine like cabernet or merlot, 3 cloves of crushed garlic, 2 tablespoons of fresh thyme or rosemary, and 1 teaspoon of black pepper.

65

IF YOU FEAR PUBLIC SPEAKING the way Paris Hilton fears obscurity, then you might think you shouldn't eat anything before a presentation lest it land on the people in the front row. You're worrying for nothing. Before your speech, have a cup of yogurt and a handful of nuts. Scientists in Slovakia gave people 3 grams each of two amino acids—lysine and arginine—or a placebo and asked them to deliver a speech. Blood measurements of stress hormones revealed that the amino-acid-fortified guys were half as anxious during and after the speech as those who took the placebo. Yogurt is one of the best food sources of lysine; nuts, of arginine.

66

HERE'S THE THING about food labels: They're essentially fun-house mirrors because they can paint a distorted picture of what's actually inside. A serving isn't necessarily the whole package but, often, only a fraction of it. Use these handy guidelines to help you gauge how much you're actually eating.

▶ Two fingers: one serving of cheese

▶ Open palm: one serving of meat

▶ Closed fist: one serving of fruit or vegetables

▶ Cupped hand: one serving of cereal or grain

▶ Tip of thumb: one serving of margarine, oil, or salad dressing

▶ Thumb: one serving of candy

67

BESIDES YOUR BILLS, your blender, and dried-up milk puddles, you should keep an avocado on your kitchen counter. Add a slice to a sandwich. It adds not only monounsaturated and polyunsaturated fats but also potassium, folate, and fiber.

68

TO MOST PEOPLE, coconut is about as much of a health food as a chili dog. Even though coconut has loads of saturated fat, you can occasionally have some as a snack. More than

50 percent of its saturated fat content is lauric acid, which boosts good HDL cholesterol (as well as the bad LDL kind). The rest of that fat is made up of what's called medium-chain fatty acids, which have no effect on cholesterol. Have a handful of shredded, unsweetened coconut, but don't gorge; it is indeed high in calories.

69

IN AN ERA when your time is taxed more heavily than your paycheck, every minute you save buys you an extra one to spend however you like. You can shorten the grilling time of chicken by pounding the breasts to an even thickness before cooking. Put each breast between sheets of plastic, and, starting at the thickest point, pound it with a tenderizer or the heel of your hand until the thick part is even with the thin part.

70

A NICE RUB FOR SALMON: 1 tablespoon of smoked paprika, 1 teaspoon of salt, and 1 teaspoon of black pepper. Mix together and rub over salmon steaks. Squeeze a drop or two of honey on top while grilling.

71

SOME THINGS ARE BETTER dry—like ceilings and armpits—but ground beef is not one of them. Super-lean ground beef can dry out fast, but you can keep it moist with vegetables like onions, red peppers, and mushrooms. Add them raw or sauté in a little bit of oil, then mix into the meat.

72

NO CALORIES, NO FAT, sweet taste—what's not to love about diet soda? Turns out it could be the liquid equivalent of meat loaf: Drinking diet soda may actually raise your risk of getting fat. Researchers from the University of Texas Health Science Center at San Antonio compared regular- and diet-soda consumption with weight changes in 1,200 people over an 8-year period. They found that those who drank at least one diet soda every day had a 55 percent chance of becoming overweight anyway—a 22 percent lead over regular-soda drinkers. My take: Neither choice helps your efforts. Your Abs Diet beverage repertoire should be water, low-fat dairy products, tea, coffee, and an occasional cup of fruit juice or alcohol.

73

SPEAKING OF WHICH, don't reach for a soda if you're feeling sluggish at work. British researchers found that people who downed a drink with 42 milligrams of sugar and 30 milligrams of caffeine (what's in a regular 12-ounce soda) had greater lapses in attention for the next hour than those who sipped a sugar-free drink. Best option: a sugar-free drink with 80 milligrams of caffeine—which happens to be the stats of an 8-ounce cup of coffee.

74

FOR THE TIMES when fruit or a smoothie just won't do it after dinner, choose a dessert that has fewer than 100 calories and zero fat—like sorbet or Italian ice.

75

HAS YOUR STOMACH seen more sandwiches than a construction worker's lunch pail? Replace the refined-flour sandwich handles with a large leaf of romaine lettuce. Just jam lean meats and fish right into it.

76

YOU KNOW WHAT MAKES a good spaghetti sauce: garlic, oregano, a hearty meatball, and a neck-high napkin. Now make it even better: Add in wilted spinach and other veg-etables. You reduce your calorie count but still fill your belly when you eat more "free" veggies and less pasta.

77

THINK ABOUT THIS when you're doing the seventh-inning saunter over to the concession stand. People who eat 3 ounces or more of processed meats (sausage, bacon, ham, hot dogs) a day have a 15 percent greater chance of developing stomach cancer.

78

BURN YOUR FAT by burning your tongue. Overweight people are more likely to fry calories after a meal that contains chile peppers than after one that doesn't pack heat. How do we know? In a study, participants' levels of insulin—a hor-mone that signals the body to store fat—were 32 percent lower following the spicy meal. Capsaicin, the chemical that makes chile peppers hot, may improve the liver's ability to clear insulin from the bloodstream after a meal.

79

PROOF THAT you should request a to-go box with your order: In a study at the University of Arkansas, people guessing the number of calories in sample restaurant meals underes-timated by as much as 600 calories. Order a half portion of an entrée, split a meal with someone, or ask for a box and immediately cut the dish in half and stow it away.

80

I'M AS INTO MEASURING out food as O'Reilly is into liberal actors. That said, whenever you're trying to adjust your weight, it's important to keep portion sizes in mind. If you make an effort to scoop out and slurp up smaller amounts, you're going to get exponential results. Penn State researchers found that simply by taking three-quarters of their typical servings, people ate 10 percent fewer calories a day—without feeling any hungrier. One place to start is with whole-grain pasta and rice. A survey found that nearly 60 percent of people overestimate the serving sizes of those specific foods.

81

A SALAD A DAY may help you live longer, according to Louisiana State researchers. In a study of more than 17,000 people, scientists found that those who ate one serving of a garden salad daily consumed significantly more folate and vitamins B_6, C, and E than those who didn't. The amount of raw vegetables in one serving of salad is estimated to increase life span by 2 years. Take note, burger boy: Almost 70 percent of men don't eat greens daily.

82

THE BEST CHOICES at your local coffee joint typically don't involve the words *mocha, cream,* or anything *-iato* or *-accino.* If you can transition from your expensive coffee addiction to one that involves tea, you'll speed up your weight-loss efforts. When Taiwanese researchers studied more than 1,100 people over a 10-year period, they determined that those who drank black, green, or oolong tea at least once a week had 20 percent less body fat than those who drank no tea. Tea extracts seem to decrease fat absorption and blood glucose while increasing metabolic rate.

83

UNDERRATED INGREDIENT of the day, No. 1: pine nuts. Harvested in Europe, Mexico, China, and the United States, these pine-tree seeds contain plenty of healthy fat and more protein per ounce than many other nuts. Their subtle, nutty taste and crunchy texture make a perfect topping for virtually any salad, vegetable, meat, or pasta dish.

84

UNDERRATED INGREDIENT of the day, No. 2: quinoa. Although this South American seed is considered a whole grain, it's actually from the same food family as spinach and beets. And unlike wheat and rice, it provides a healthy dose of all the essential amino acids, making it a complete protein. Another bonus: It's a good source of fiber and heart-healthy omega-3 fats. Try it as an alternative side dish to rice or pasta.

85

UNDERRATED INGREDIENT of the day, No. 3: Swiss chard. It has potassium, vitamin K (for bone health), and vitamin E (an antioxidant). Chop a bunch into 1-inch pieces and sauté in olive oil with a few chopped cloves of garlic. Mix in a can of drained cannellini beans, season with salt and pepper, and serve as a bed for grilled chicken or fish.

86

IN A PINCH with a nagging sweet tooth? Chewing gum may curb your cravings. One study showed that when people chomped on sugarless gum for at least 15 minutes, first 1 hour after eating and then again at the 2-hour mark, their desire for sweets decreased by 11 percent, compared with people who didn't chew.

87

SEE NO EVIL, eat no evil. You'll eat less if you use small plates and bowls for your meals. Cornell researchers found that people dish out 50 percent more food when they have larger dishes.

88

THE BEST DISEASE-FIGHTING salad ever contains ingredients with some of the highest antioxidant levels around.

Complement your red leaf lettuce with yellow peppers, yellow onions, pecans, and red kidney beans. Drizzle with some olive oil and vinegar.

89

AND YOU THOUGHT DAIRY was the only path to the super-power nutrient calcium. Three ounces of canned salmon contains 235 milligrams of the bone-building, fat-fighting stuff.

90

ONE WAY YOU DON'T WANT to lose weight: by getting sick from the food you eat. Set your refrigerator for 40°F or colder to stop bacterial growth.

91

CRAVE FRIED CHICKEN but fear the fat? Then add a low-fat crust that still gives you crunch. A whisked egg acts like glue, holding the crust to the meat. It also gives the chicken a small protein boost. Crack open an egg in a shallow bowl, whisk it, and dip the chicken in it. Then roll the chicken in a mixture of 1 tablespoon finely grated Parmesan cheese, 1 tablespoon Italian-style bread crumbs, and a pinch of black pepper. Another option: Roll the coated chicken in ⅓ cup of your favorite nuts. Then bake it rather than frying it, for a crisp crust.

92

WHILE YOU MAY BE well versed in inspecting fruits and melons, here's a tip for vegetable viability. With asparagus, broccoli, and cauliflower, the tighter the buds are closed, the fresher the produce. Feel free to use as cocktail-party fodder or a pickup line in the produce section. You're welcome.

93

A MICROWAVE WORKS FINE for boiling water, nuking morning eggs, or splitting turkey dogs, but don't discount the power of the Crock-Pot. Taiwanese scientists found that a traditional Chinese cooking method—simmering meat slowly for hours in a soy sauce marinade—makes pork healthier by reducing the number of cholesterol oxidation products, chemicals that form when the meat is cooked and may increase cancer risk.

94

YOU DON'T HAVE TO BE a lunch-toting toddler to idolize the almighty PB&J. Eating foods rich in magnesium, such as peanut butter and whole-wheat bread, can protect your heart, according to a University of Virginia study. Their 15-year study of 7,000 men showed double the risk of coronary heart disease among those who were magnesium deficient. Just make sure your sandwich consists of whole-grain bread, all-natural peanut butter, and fresh berries.

95

CHOCOLATE IS BAD when attached to a cone or any phrase including "death by," but it's not always the evil ingredient it's made out to be. In fact, pure cocoa has more antioxidants than green tea, according to Cornell research.

96

HERE'S ONE TIME when getting a C is better than average: Arizona State researchers found that people who take 500 milligrams of vitamin C daily burn 39 percent more fat during exercise than those who ingest only small amounts of the nutrient. Researchers suspect that low levels of C impede the body's ability to use fat as energy. Most guys don't get enough, so you may want to try a supplement.

97

MAYBE MULTICHEESE LASAGNA isn't the way to get it, but don't give up on ricotta cheese. Researchers found that people who ate a daily 2.8 grams of whey (the liquid in ricotta cheese) produced fewer stress hormones. They also had 48 percent more tryptophan, the substance that tells your body to release more of the feel-good chemical serotonin. A cool way to get it:

Turkey Lasagna

½   pound turkey sausage, casings removed
2   large yellow onions, chopped
2   teaspoons oregano
2   cans (14 ounces each) diced tomatoes
3   cups nonfat ricotta cheese
1   cup grated Parmesan cheese
9   whole-wheat lasagna noodles, cooked

Preheat the oven to 350°F.

Quickly fry the sausage, onions, and oregano. Stir in the tomatoes. In a bowl, combine the ricotta and ½ cup of the Parmesan. Spread a third of the tomato/meat mixture in a lightly oiled 9" × 13" baking dish. Arrange three noodles in the dish and spread with half of the cheese mixture. Repeat these layers. Top with the last layer of noodles, the remaining third of the tomato-meat mixture, and the remaining ½ cup Parmesan. Cover with foil and bake for 45 minutes. Remove the foil and bake for 15 minutes more. Let stand 15 to 20 minutes before serving.

Makes 6 servings

Per serving: 372 calories, 29 g protein, 40 g carbohydrates, 12 g fat (29% of calories)

98

JAZZ UP A BLAND TURKEY WRAP with hummus. The ground-chickpea-and-sesame spread has protein, fiber, and only 1½ grams of fat per tablespoonful.

99

IN THE MASTER-OF-MY-GRILL category, try this: Marinate your chicken with 2 tablespoons orange juice, 1 tablespoon hoisin sauce, and ¼ teaspoon red-pepper flakes. Just mix the ingredients in a resealable plastic bag, drop in the chicken, seal, shake, and refrigerate for an hour. Make a little extra marinade (the stuff used for soaking harbors bacteria and should be discarded), and brush it on the chicken while cooking, to keep it moist.

Chapter 4

A SECOND HELPING OF SECRETS
More Nutrition News You Can Use

MOST DIETS GIVE the same warning about second helpings that fathers give about their teenage daughters—don't even think about touching them, or there'll be hell to pay. On the Abs Diet, it's okay to have under-control second helpings, provided they're Powerfood-packed. In that spirit, I'm going to serve up another 49 secrets to help you control cravings, eat smart, and make nutrition decisions that will put you on the right path to a lean and strong body. Get yourself a clean plate, and help yourself to this buffet of information and inspiration.

1

WHY I LIKE TO SUB in a second slice of meat for a potato: Australian scientists found that replacing some of the carbohydrates in your diet with red meat can lower blood pressure. In the study, hypertensive men and women exchanged 8 percent of their daily calories from bread, cereal, potatoes, or pasta with an equal amount of lean red meat. As a result, their systolic blood pressure dropped four points in just 8 weeks. Credit arginine—an amino acid in red meat, which may help dilate blood vessels—with lowering blood pressure.

2

YOU'VE SPENT ENOUGH late nights and early mornings slaving over projects and nasty move-your-butt e-mails from bosses to have a pretty intimate relationship with caffeine. But how well do you know your liquid boosters? To determine how much of a jolt you can expect from popular beverages, University of Florida researchers analyzed 36 widely available drinks. Here are some milligrams of caffeine per ounce comparisons, so you can see which drinks pack the most punch.

ENERGY DRINK

SoBe Adrenaline Rush, 76.7 milligrams per 8.3 ounces; 9.2 milligrams per ounce

BOTTLED TEA

Nestea Cool Lemon Iced Tea, 11.5 milligrams per 12 ounces; 0.96 milligram per ounce

READY-TO-DRINK COFFEE

Starbucks Doubleshot, 105.7 milligrams per 6.5 ounces; 16.3 milligrams per ounce

DIET SODA

Diet Coke with Lime, 39.6 milligrams per 12 ounces; 3.3 milligrams per ounce

BLACK COFFEE

Dunkin' Donuts regular, 143 milligrams per 16 ounces; 8.9 milligrams per ounce

REGULAR SODA

Mountain Dew, 45.4 milligrams per 12 ounces; 3.8 milligrams per ounce

3

SCARY FACT OF THE DAY: Ninety-six percent of men don't eat the recommended nine servings of fruits and vegetables a day.

4

WHEN IT COMES TO OIL for your car, you generally don't give it a whole lot of thought. Different story if you're cooking up fish, chicken, or vegetables. The worst oils: those high in saturated fats, like coconut oil and lard. The best: olive, safflower, and canola oils, which are high in monounsaturated and poly-unsaturated fats. See the table at the bottom of this page.

5

HERE'S A BREAD to pack your turkey into: organic 100 percent whole-grain flourless stuff. It's made with fresh grains and legumes, such as wheat, barley, beans, spelt, and millet, that are first allowed to sprout. Then the sprouts are formed into batches of dough and slowly baked. Sprouted-grain bread has more protein, fiber, and B vitamins than loaves made with refined flour, according to researchers in India. Plus, each slice is certified as low-glycemic, which helps reduce your risk of developing heart disease. Look for it in the freezer aisle. Because it has no preservatives, it must be kept frozen until sold.

OIL	SERVING SIZE	CALORIES	TOTAL FAT (G)
Olive oil	1 Tbsp	119	13.5
Safflower oil	1 Tbsp	120	13.6
Canola oil	1 Tbsp	124	14.0
Corn oil	1 Tbsp	120	13.6
Peanut oil	1 Tbsp	119	13.5
Palm oil	1 Tbsp	120	13.6
Margarine	2 tsp	67	7.6
Butter	2 tsp	68	7.7
Coconut oil	1 Tbsp	120	13.6
Lard	1 Tbsp	115	12.8

6

SOME HEALTH FOODS are nothing but impostors. They look like they're good for you but aren't. One culprit: rice cakes, which have one of the highest glycemic-index values of any food. That means they raise blood-sugar and insulin levels faster and higher than table sugar or white bread. As a result, your body starts storing fat instead of burning it.

7

BEFORE BED, here's what to watch out for (besides bad Jimmy Kimmel jokes): protein, which supplies the brain with the amino acid tyrosine, which boosts alertness. Plus, some of those high-protein foods may also be high in fat, which digests slowly and makes sleep more fitful. Better choice: carbs, which provide tryptophan, the sleep-inducing amino acid.

8

WHEN IT COMES TO BOOZE, you know how much trouble you can get into—and you have the mug shot to prove it. Here's

SATURATED FAT (G)	MONOUNSATURATED FAT (G)	POLYUNSATURATED FAT (G)
1.8	10.0	1.2
1.2	1.7	10.1
1.0	8.3	4.1
1.7	3.3	7.9
2.3	6.2	4.3
6.7	5.0	1.3
1.3	2.7	3.3
4.8	2.2	0.3
11.8	0.8	0.2
5.0	5.8	1.4

another good reason to avoid those lost weekends, though: Binge drinking may lead to increased belly fat. Researchers at the University at Buffalo in New York found that, compared with those who down more than four drinks at a time once or twice every 2 weeks, men who drank the same amount but in smaller daily doses had lower levels of abdominal fat.

9

CRAVING SWEETS but fear the repercussions of a Cold Stone run? Have a Tootsie Pop. It's long-lasting and low-calorie to help take the edge off.

10

I CERTAINLY UNDERSTAND if your mornings have heavier traffic than the Atlanta airport. But if you can, you may want to schedule your workouts for first thing. Scientists at Syracuse University in New York recently found that a single weight-training session reduces the effect of a high-sugar meal on blood glucose by 15 percent for more than 12 hours after a workout. Why? Exercise drains your muscles' fuel reserves—stored glucose known as glycogen. To ensure that you have plenty of energy for your next workout, your body immediately shuttles any available glucose to your muscles, where it's packed away for future use—helping to reduce blood-glucose levels. Until glycogen levels are replenished, which can take several hours, high-sugar foods aren't as detrimental—so make sure the benefit applies while you're awake and eating.

11

IF YOU'RE HAVING TROUBLE falling asleep and you're just twisting and turning instead, eat a couple of handfuls of cherries an hour before bed. Researchers at the University of Texas found that tart cherries are one of the best natural sources of melatonin, a popular over-the-counter sleep aid. You can keep the pits off the sheets by drinking juices

made with cherry concentrate; they have 10 times the melatonin content of the fruit.

12

THE PROLIFERATION OF ALL THOSE little pink, blue, and yellow
packets probably has you wondering which sugar substitute
is the best choice. Here's the lowdown on the more popular
crystals.

SACCHARIN (SWEET'N LOW)
What it is: product of a reaction between sulfur dioxide,
chlorine, ammonia, and two biochemical acids; in Crest and
Colgate
Calories: ⅛ calorie per teaspoon
Flavor profile: metallic and bitter aftertaste; 300 to
500 times sweeter than sugar
Possible side effects: linked to cancer in rats but not
in humans; FDA removed warning labels

ASPARTAME (NUTRASWEET, EQUAL)
What it is: combination of two amino acids, aspartic
acid and phenylalanine; in Diet Coke, Diet Pepsi, and most
other diet sodas
Calories: zero
Flavor profile: distinctly chemical; 180 times sweeter
than sugar
Possible side effects: none, unless you have a rare
genetic condition called phenylketonuria (PKU), in which
your body can't process phenylalanine

SUCRALOSE (SPLENDA)
What it is: sugar molecules blended with chlorine; in
Arizona brand diet iced teas
Calories: zero
Flavor profile: slightly chemical; 600 times sweeter
than sugar
Possible side effects: none

SUGAR ALCOHOLS

What it is: sugar molecules with added hydrogen; in Hershey's low-carb chocolate bars

Calories: ¾ the calories of sugar

Flavor profile: none; same sweetness as sugar, but less impact on blood sugar

Possible side effects: bloating, gas, diarrhea

STEVIA

What it is: dried leaves of the stevia plant; not yet FDA approved for use in food

Calories: zero

Flavor profile: licorice-like; 150 to 400 times sweeter than sugar

Possible side effects: not yet known; no clinical trials conducted

13

THOUGH STEREOTYPED as the choice of the pregnant set, pickles can aid your weight-loss efforts. Order extra on sandwiches, and begin any high-carbohydrate meal with a side salad that's mixed with a vinegar-based dressing, such as balsamic vinaigrette or Italian. Remember the Swedes who ate white bread and vinegar (page 29)? They felt fuller thanks to acetic acid, a primary component of vinegar, dressings—and pickled products.

14

CRAVING GRILLED CHEESE with the same ferocity with which a child wills a snow day? Here's the recipe, minus all the saturated fat in the typical version: Use whole-wheat bread and part-skim mozzarella. Crisp it in a skillet moistened with a little olive oil. To protect your prostate, add a couple of lycopene-packed tomato slices. If you need longer-lasting satisfaction, throw in a slice or two of lean ham to jack up the protein count, keeping your appetite in check.

15

GO AHEAD and make the obligatory baked bean joke. Done? Now, tasty as they are, baked beans are typically loaded with saturated fat. Instead, put together this sweet concoction.

½   cup ketchup
1   bottle (12 ounces) black-cherry soda
2   tablespoons spicy brown mustard
2   teaspoons apple-cider vinegar
⅛   teaspoon ground black pepper
3   cans (15 ounces each) beans (black, pinto, or kidney), rinsed and drained
5   slices turkey bacon

Dump everything except the beans and bacon into a 2-quart microwaveable dish and mix well. Stir in the beans. Cover tightly with plastic wrap and nuke, stirring every 5 minutes or so, for 15 to 18 minutes, or until the liquid thickens. While that's heating, cut each bacon strip into 4 equal pieces. Uncover the beans and put the bacon on top in a single layer. Microwave, uncovered, for 5 to 7 minutes, or until the bacon is cooked and crispy around the edges.

Makes 6 servings

Per serving: 253 calories, 14 g protein, 37 g carbohydrates, 6 g fat (1 g saturated), 10 g fiber, 1,011 mg sodium

16

POP A KIWI into your smoothie. Scientists at the University of Oslo recently determined that eating kiwifruit may cut your risk of a heart attack.

17

FIND YOURSELF in the awkward position of showing up to work with a black eye? Skip the shades and eat a papaya. A black eye, like any other bruise, is caused by blood from ruptured vessels trapped under the skin. An enzyme found in papaya changes the blood's molecular structure so it's more easily absorbed by the body.

18

YOU MAY BE ABLE to curtail your eating by doing more than duct taping your mouth. Eat more foods rich in zinc. In a study published in the *Journal of the American College of Nutrition*, researchers found that consuming more of the mineral caused a rise in leptin, a hormone that controls body fat by telling you when you've had enough to eat. Your body takes an increase in leptin as a signal to build muscle instead of store fat. Lean red meats and whole grains are rich in zinc.

19

WHEN YOU'RE BOILING corn on the cob, add some ground red pepper to the water for butter-free Cajun corn.

20

TO GET THE MOST fiber from canned beans, don't drain away the liquid.

21

UNLIKE FOODS IN PACKAGES and friends who borrow your couch, fresh vegetables don't come with expiration dates. Rule of thumb: The more water a vegetable contains, the less time it will last. Here's a guide to length of freshness.

LONG (A WEEK OR MORE)

Broccoli
Cabbage
Cooking greens (chard, kale, mustard greens)

Hard squash (butternut)*

Lettuce and salad greens (romaine, iceberg, endive, radicchio)

Root vegetables (beets, turnips, carrots, radishes)

MEDIUM (4–5 DAYS)

Asparagus

Cauliflower

Eggplant

Green beans

Green bell peppers

Lettuce (Boston butter, soft head, green leaf)

Mushrooms

Scallions

Spinach

Sweet onions

SHORT (1–3 DAYS)

Avocados

Corn

Cucumbers

Herbs (basil, oregano, sage)

Lettuce and salad greens (arugula, spring mix, red leaf lettuces)

Red or yellow bell peppers

Tomatoes

Yellow summer squash

Zucchini

*Some hard winter squashes can last up to 3 months.

22

BESIDES ITS EFFECTIVENESS in decreasing cancer risk and aiding weight loss, green tea also sweetens bad breath. In a Canadian study comparing green tea with the mouth-freshening powers of mint, parsley, and chewing gum, the tea emerged as the most effective killer of the bacteria that cause your breath to stink.

23

MAYBE A BLENDER got you into this mess in the first place, but now you can use it to make a smoothie that will ease your hangover and help you avoid alcohol-induced dehydration. It's loaded with vitamin C to help combat binge-related cell damage, and the fructose in the fruit juices helps speed the metabolism of liquor. Upset stomach? The ginger in ginger ale will help quell the motion sickness caused by your spinning bedroom. And the acidophilus bacteria in the yogurt may help get your gut back in chemical balance.

1   cup tangerine/orange blended juice
1   tablespoon lime juice
½   cup low-fat vanilla yogurt
½   cup Canada Dry ginger ale (or any ginger ale that
      contains real ginger)
Sprig of mint

In a blender, combine the tangerine/orange juice, lime juice, yogurt, and ginger ale. Blend until smooth. Garnish with the mint.

246 calories, 4.6 g protein, 53.7 g carbohydrates, 2.3 g fat (8.4% of calories), 0 g fiber

24

SALT MAY BE GREAT in oceans, with margaritas, and after a sweat-soaked workout. But it's easy to take in 7,000 milligrams a day without trying. Too much can not only raise blood pressure and weaken bones but cause kidney stones. Watch out for stealth sources, like chicken: Salt solutions are pumped into poultry parts to plump them up. Check labels, and look for chicken that doesn't come with added broth.

25

IF RUNNING GIVES YOU nighttime calf cramps, drink tonic water before bed. It contains quinine, a plant extract that acts as a muscle relaxant. Add lemon or mix with orange juice to reduce the tonic water's bitterness.

26

LOTS OF GREAT THINGS come in red—sports cars and lingerie come to mind. So do foods like kidney beans, red beans, and apples. These low-glycemic carbohydrates don't cause insulin spikes during digestion.

27

BUY FISH TUESDAY THROUGH FRIDAY. Many markets get their fish on Tuesday, Wednesday, and Thursday, so if you wait until Sunday or Monday, you'll get the week's leftovers.

28

THE YEAR IS FILLED with endless diet-busting occasions. One of the biggest: the night your costumed kid comes home with a sack full of sin. If you must go five fingers into his bag after your Power Ranger goes to bed on Halloween, choose these bite-size bits that have less than 1.5 grams of fat per piece.

Twizzlers (11 grams, or 1 stick): 36 calories; 0 grams fat; 3.3 calories per gram

Candy corn (10 grams, or 10 pieces): 63 calories; 0 grams fat; 6.3 calories per gram

Smarties (28 grams, or 1 roll of 15 pieces): 100 calories; 0 grams fat; 3.6 calories per gram

Tootsie Roll (6.6 grams, or 1 piece): 27 calories; 0.5 gram fat; 4 calories per gram

3 Musketeers (5.8 grams): 24 calories; 0.7 gram fat; 4.1 calories per gram

York Peppermint Pattie (13.6 grams): 53 calories; 1 gram fat; 3.9 calories per gram

Milky Way (8.6 grams): 38 calories; 1.4 grams fat; 4.4 calories per gram

29

GOOD-FOR-YOU TUNA can quickly become a diet disaster with the wrong dressing. Instead of fatty mayo, stir a squeeze of lemon juice, a dash of pepper, and a few drops of hot pepper sauce into your tuna.

30

SIMULATE A REUBEN by replacing fatty corned beef with turkey ham and topping it with low-fat mozzarella, mustard, spicy shredded cabbage, and pickles. Slap it all on traditional rye bread and broil until the cheese melts.

31

THE DARKER AND RICHER YOUR CHOCOLATE, the more of the feel-good chemicals called endorphins your body will produce.

32

AN ODE TO APRICOTS: They're a good source of fiber and packed with vitamin A. And you can eat as many as you want: One fresh apricot contains a mere 17 calories (a half cup of dried ones contains 155).

33

DON'T BE CONNED by sneaky tricks that restaurants use to get you to buy more—and thus eat more. One study found that people order more desserts when the foods are described with ethnic names.

34

COOL CHICKEN FACT: White meat contains one-third less fat than dark.

35

A USDA STUDY found that men don't get the recommended daily amounts of every nutrient they need. Here's what to aim for and (in parentheses) what the average man gets.

Calcium: 1,000 milligrams (879)

Magnesium: 410 milligrams (321)

Phosphorus: 700 milligrams (1,459)

Folate: 400 micrograms (303)

Niacin: 16 milligrams (26.9)

Riboflavin: 1.3 milligrams (2.3)

Thiamin: 1.2 milligrams (1.9)

Vitamin B_6: 1.3 milligrams (2.1)

Vitamin B_{12}: 2.4 micrograms (6.6)

Vitamin C: 90 milligrams (106)

Vitamin E: 15 milligrams (9.8)

36

NOT THAT I'M SUGGESTING you ditch your toothpaste, but some foods are also natural teeth cleaners. For example:

▶ An ounce of low-fat cheese can neutralize cavity-causing acids.

▶ Fiber in apples and other crunchy vegetables can wipe away plaque.

▶ Salsa or jalapeño peppers make your mouth water, which helps neutralize acids.

▶ Nonfat yogurt helps fortify bone that builds strong teeth.

37

INSTEAD OF A PROTEIN BAR before a workout, try dried figs (to eat, not to wear, Tarzan). Figs have slow-burning energy to help get you through a workout. Afterward, reach for a glass of chocolate milk. A University of Washington study found that drinks that blend carbohydrates and protein, such as chocolate milk, are nearly 40 percent more effective than protein alone at helping your muscles repair themselves and grow after a workout.

38

AIOLI—A LIGHT SAUCE that's made of olive oil, eggs, and garlic—is a good substitute for mayo because of the healthy ingredients. Though not many supermarkets stock it, you can find it at gourmet stores or order it online.

39

IF YOU'RE LOOKING to find someone to join you in the parent-to-be process, snack on celery. It's packed with androstenone and androstenol, two pheromones that play a big role in attraction.

40

BEEF JERKY IS HIGH in protein and doesn't raise insulin levels. While some brands are packed with high-sodium ingredients, such as MSG and sodium nitrate, chemical-free products are available. Gourmet natural beef jerky, for example, has no preservatives and is made from lean, grass-fed beef that, unlike grain-fed products, contains the same healthy omega-3 fats found in fish.

41

LIMA BEANS are the best vegetable source of potassium, plus they're high in iron, B vitamins, and calcium.

42

PECANS CONTAIN SOME OF THE HIGHEST AMOUNTS of disease-fighting antioxidants, according to a USDA study.

43

HERE'S WHY BEER-LEAGUE SOFTBALL PLAYERS have bellies bigger than domed stadiums: Within seconds of swigging a sip, beer passes through your esophagus and into your stomach. About 20 percent of the alcohol is absorbed into your bloodstream; the rest is absorbed from your intestines. The alcohol travels through your blood to your liver, where it's broken down. During this process, waste products called acetate and acetaldehyde are created. They signal your body to stop burning fat. At the same time, your body starts making fat from another waste product of alcohol, acetyl-CoA. Your body can effectively process only 0.5 to 1 ounce of alcohol per hour (a 12-ounce beer contains 0.6 ounce of alcohol), so the more you drink, the longer your body is inhibited from burning fat, and the more fat builds up from the excess acetyl-CoA.

44

TRYING TO BE A PAPA? Make Brazil nuts your nut of choice. They're a top source of selenium, a vitamin that keeps your sperm cells healthy.

45

YOU DON'T HAVE TO BE A CELEBRITY CHEF to cook like one. Here's a unique and easy salsa recipe from Bobby Flay: Start with a base of 2 cups of either chopped tomatoes, mangoes, papayas, pineapple, or roasted tomatillos. Add a handful of chopped cilantro, some chopped red onion, a finely diced jalapeño chile pepper, fresh lime juice, and salt and pepper. Use fruit salsas with fish, tomato salsas with steak and lamb.

46

TO MAKE EGGS MORE INTERESTING, stir in tomatoes and cilantro after you scramble them.

47

HAVE WHOLE-GRAIN TOAST with your eggs. A study showed that those who ate a 400-calorie breakfast with carbohydrates worked out nearly half an hour longer than those who skipped breakfast.

48

FENNEL, a crunchy, sweet vegetable with a mild licorice flavor, is chock-full of vitamin C, fiber, and antioxidants. To prepare it, remove the long stems and cut off the core at the base of the bulb. Quarter the bulb and sauté it with a bit of olive oil in a pan over medium heat. After 5 minutes, turn the heat to low and add ½ cup of orange juice. Cover and simmer for 10 minutes, or until it's soft. Goes best with fish or chicken.

49

PICKING THE RIGHT FOODS is half the battle when it comes to eating well, so use these mental tricks from *Men's Health* magazine mental guru Marc Salem to help you make the best decisions along the way.

Drink up. Since we often interpret thirst as hunger, reach for a glass of ice water every time you feel hungry, and you'll eat less.

Pinch your nostrils or earlobes for 10 seconds. These acupressure points will help hunger pass.

Use bright lights. Dim lights lower inhibitions, so eat in bright lights, whether on the couch or in the kitchen.

Don't eat during meetings. You're more likely to munch mindlessly during intense discussions. Have a cup of coffee, rather than trying to negotiate a deal over a meal.

Stop touching so much. You're more likely to buy something once you touch it (that's why marketers have cool, colorful packaging). Keep your hands off anything in the junk-food aisles, and it's more likely to stay on the shelf.

Chapter 5

THE 100 BEST FOODS EVER
Our Ranking, Your Menu

YOU ALREADY KNOW how I feel: Eating the literally hundreds of different foods that fall into the 12 categories of Powerfoods is all you need to do in order to change your belly and body forever. Mixing up those foods will give you an ideal combination of protein, carbohydrates, healthy fat, fiber, and other important nutrients. That said, as Letterman and *Billboard* have taught us, there's a lot of insight that can be gained from looking at ranking systems.

The following ranking, vetted by *Men's Health* weight-loss coach Heidi Skolnick, MS, CDN, FACSM, outlines the 100 very best foods you can have (most will fall into Powerfood categories, of course). This list is based not only on calorie counts and other nutrients, like protein and fiber, but also on vitamins and disease-fighting substances. Like any good ranking, you can argue about the order all you want—as long as you're eating these foods while you're doing so.

About the Chart

Most of the following foods are low-cholesterol, low-sodium, and trans fat–free, as well as low-calorie. All fruits and vegetables, of course, are loaded with nutrients. Some foods have very small amounts of certain nutrients—too little to really measure (did you know that vegetables even have protein?). This chart highlights the nutrients that are primarily packed into these specific foods.

Protein: satiating and muscle-building

Fiber: heart-healthy; keeps you full and satisfied so you don't overeat

Whole grains: unrefined carbohydrates loaded with fiber

Healthy fats: unsaturated fats that help unclog arteries and fill you up

Calcium: bone-building mineral also shown to promote weight loss

Other minerals: nutrients needed in small amounts to help your body function

Vitamins: key nutrients for growth and to help fight disease

Polyphenols: antioxidants shown to reduce risks of heart disease and cancer

Flavonoids: plant compounds that work like disease-fighting antioxidants

Make these 100 foods part of your regular shopping list, and integrate them into your meals at every opportunity.

RANKING	FOOD	PROTEIN	FIBER	WHOLE GRAINS	HEALTHY FATS	
1	Berries (raspberries, blueberries, strawberries)		✓			
2	Eggs	✓				
3	Low-fat yogurt	✓				
4	Black beans	✓	✓			
5	Kiwifruit		✓			
6	Almonds	✓			✓	
7	Quinoa (nutty grain similar to rice or couscous)	✓	✓	✓	✓	
8	Salmon	✓			✓	

CALCIUM	OTHER MINERALS	VITAMINS	POLYPHENOLS	FLAVONOIDS
	Manganese, magnesium, potassium, copper	A, B, C, E	✓	✓
	Selenium, iodine, molybdenum, phosphorus	A, B, D, E		
✓	Iodine, phosphorus, potassium, molybdenum, zinc	B		
	Molybdenum, manganese, magnesium, phosphorus, iron	B	✓	✓
	Magnesium, potassium, copper, manganese, phosphorus	C, E	✓	
	Manganese, magnesium, potassium, copper, phosphorus	B, E		✓
	Manganese, magnesium, iron, copper, phosphorus	B		
	Selenium, phosphorus, magnesium	B, D, E		

RANKING	FOOD	PROTEIN	FIBER	WHOLE GRAINS	HEALTHY FATS	
9	Oats and oatmeal	✓	✓	✓		
10	Spinach and kale	✓	✓			
11	Mango					
12	Tomatoes					
13	Cantaloupe					
14	Turkey	✓				
15	Olive oil				✓	
16	Broccoli		✓			

CALCIUM	OTHER MINERALS	VITAMINS	POLYPHENOLS	FLAVONOIDS
	Manganese, selenium, phosphorus, magnesium	B		
✓	Manganese, magnesium, iron, potassium, copper, phosphorus, zinc, selenium	A, B, C, K		
	Potassium, phosphorus, magnesium	A, B, C, E		
	Molybdenum, potassium, manganese, chromium, copper, magnesium, iron, phosphorus	A, B, C, E, K		✓
	Potassium	A, B, C	✓	
	Iron, zinc, potassium, selenium, phosphorus	B		
		E	✓	
✓	Manganese, potassium, phosphorus, magnesium, iron, zinc	A, B, C, E, K	✓	✓

RANKING	FOOD	PROTEIN	FIBER	WHOLE GRAINS	HEALTHY FATS	
17	Barley		✓	✓		
18	Avocado		✓		✓	
19	Sweet potato		✓			
20	Wheat germ	✓	✓	✓	✓	
21	Walnuts	✓			✓	
22	Citrus fruits (oranges, lemons, grapefruit)		✓			
23	Soybeans (edamame)	✓	✓		✓	
24	Mushrooms		✓			
25	Apricots		✓			
26	Peanut butter, all natural	✓	✓		✓	

CALCIUM	OTHER MINERALS	VITAMINS	POLYPHENOLS	FLAVONOIDS
	Selenium, copper, manganese, phosphorus	B, E		
	Potassium, copper	B, C, K		
	Manganese, copper, potassium, iron	A, B, C		
	Potassium, iron	B, E		
	Manganese, copper			
	Calcium, potassium	A, B, C		✓
	Manganese, iron, phosphorus, magnesium, copper, potassium	B, K		✓
	Selenium, copper, potassium, phosphorus, niacin, pantothenic acid, iron	B	✓	
	Potassium	A, C		✓
	Potassium, iron	B, E		

RANKING	FOOD	PROTEIN	FIBER	WHOLE GRAINS	HEALTHY FATS	
27	Grape juice					
28	1% milk	✓				
29	Cloves					
30	Oregano					
31	Brussels sprouts	✓	✓		✓	
32	Pecans	✓			✓	
33	Turnip greens	✓	✓		✓	
34	Butternut squash		✓		✓	
35	Green tea					
36	Bananas					
37	Prunes		✓			

CALCIUM	OTHER MINERALS	VITAMINS	POLYPHENOLS	FLAVONOIDS
	Manganese, potassium	B, C	✓	✓
✓	Iodine, phosphorus, potassium	A, B, D, K		
✓	Manganese, magnesium	C, K		
✓	Iron, manganese	A, C, K		
✓	Manganese, potassium, iron, phosphorus, magnesium, copper	A, B, C, E, K		
✓	Potassium, phosphorus, magnesium, zinc	A, B, E		
✓	Manganese, potassium, magnesium, iron, phosphorus	A, B, C, K		
	Potassium, manganese, copper	A, B, C		
			✓	
	Potassium, manganese	B, C		
	Potassium, copper	A		

RANKING	FOOD	PROTEIN	FIBER	WHOLE GRAINS	HEALTHY FATS	
38	Red grapes		✓			
39	Blackstrap molasses (thick sweetener that, unlike other sweeteners, contains many nutrients)					
40	Ginger					
41	Pumpkin seeds	✓	✓		✓	
42	Sardines	✓			✓	
43	Chicken, skinless	✓			✓	
44	Seaweed (wakame, nori, kombu, laver)	✓	✓			
45	Carrots		✓			
46	Venison	✓				

CALCIUM	OTHER MINERALS	VITAMINS	POLYPHENOLS	FLAVONOIDS
	Potassium, manganese	B		✓
✓	Manganese, copper, iron, potassium, magnesium, selenium	B		
	Potassium, magnesium, copper, manganese	B, C		
	Magnesium, manganese, phosphorus, iron, copper, zinc	K		
✓	Phosphorus	D, E		
	Phosphorus, selenium	B		
✓	Zinc, iodine, iron	A, C		
	Potassium, manganese, molybdenum, phosphorus, magnesium	A, B, C, K		
	Iron, phosphorus, selenium, zinc, copper	B		

RANKING	FOOD	PROTEIN	FIBER	WHOLE GRAINS	HEALTHY FATS	
47	Beets		✓			
48	Sea vegetables (kelp, sea lettuce, dulce)	✓	✓			
49	Lean beef	✓				
50	Swiss chard	✓	✓			
51	Herring	✓			✓	
52	Turmeric					
53	Cabbage	✓	✓			
54	Parsley		✓			
55	Olives				✓	
56	Tahini (sesame seed paste)	✓	✓		✓	

CALCIUM	OTHER MINERALS	VITAMINS	POLYPHENOLS	FLAVONOIDS
	Manganese, potassium, magnesium, iron, copper, phosphorus	B, C		
✓	Iodine, magnesium, iron	B, K		
	Zinc, selenium, phosphorus, iron	B		
✓	Zinc, phosphorus, copper, manganese, magnesium, potassium	A, B, C, E, K		
✓	Iodine, selenium	A, B, D		
	Manganese, iron, potassium	B		
✓	Manganese, potassium, magnesium	A, B, K	✓	✓
	Iron	A, C, K	✓	✓
	Copper, iron	E		
✓	Manganese, copper, calcium, magnesium, iron, phosphorus, zinc	B		

RANKING	FOOD	PROTEIN	FIBER	WHOLE GRAINS	HEALTHY FATS	
57	Mustard greens	✓	✓			
58	Trout	✓				
59	Red bell peppers		✓			
60	Cherries		✓			
61	Artichokes					
62	Bok choy		✓			
63	Cauliflower		✓			
64	Figs		✓			
65	Pumpkin		✓			
66	Arugula		✓			

CALCIUM	OTHER MINERALS	VITAMINS	POLYPHENOLS	FLAVONOIDS
✓	Manganese, potassium, copper, phosphorus, iron, magnesium	A, B, C, E, K		
✓	Selenium, phosphorus	B, D		
	Molybdenum, manganese, potassium, copper	A, B, C, K		✓
	Potassium, magnesium, iron	A, B, C, E	✓	
	Potassium, iron, phosphorus	B, C		
✓	Potassium	A, B, C		
	Magnesium, phosphorus, potassium, manganese	B, C, K		
	Potassium, manganese	A, B, C, K		
	Iron, magnesium, potassium, zinc, selenium, niacin	A, B, C, E		
✓	Zinc, copper, folate, iron, magnesium, phosphorus, potassium, manganese	A, B, C, K		

RANKING	FOOD	PROTEIN	FIBER	WHOLE GRAINS	HEALTHY FATS	
67	Brown rice		✓	✓		
68	Buckwheat	✓	✓	✓		
69	Radishes		✓			
70	Watermelon					
71	Halibut	✓			✓	
72	Turnips		✓			
73	Romaine lettuce		✓			
74	Watercress					
75	Collard greens		✓			

CALCIUM	OTHER MINERALS	VITAMINS	POLYPHENOLS	FLAVONOIDS
	Manganese, selenium, magnesium, iron	B, E, K		
	Iron, magnesium, manganese	B, E, K		
✓	Iron, potassium	C		
	Potassium, magnesium	A, B, C, E		
	Copper, iron, magnesium, manganese, molybdenum, phosphorus, selenium, zinc	A, B, D, E		
✓	Copper, iron, magnesium, manganese, phosphorus, selenium, sodium, zinc	A, B, C, E, K		
	Copper, iodine, iron, magnesium, manganese, molybdenum, phosphorus, selenium, zinc	A, B, C, E, K		
✓		A, C		
✓	Calcium, copper, iron, magnesium, manganese, phosphorus, selenium, zinc	A, B, C, E, K		

RANKING	FOOD	PROTEIN	FIBER	WHOLE GRAINS	HEALTHY FATS	
76	Mustard		✓			
77	Whole-grain bread		✓	✓		
78	Soy milk, fortified	✓			✓	
79	Raisins					
80	Shrimp	✓				
81	Fennel		✓			
82	Rosemary					
83	Spelt (nutlike grain)	✓	✓	✓	✓	
84	Celery		✓			

CALCIUM	OTHER MINERALS	VITAMINS	POLYPHENOLS	FLAVONOIDS
	Iron, magnesium			
	Iron	B		
✓	Iron	A, C		
	Copper, iron, magnesium, manganese, phosphorus, selenium, zinc	A, B, C, E, K	✓	
	Copper, iron, magnesium, manganese, phosphorus, selenium, zinc	A, B, C, D, E, K		
✓	Copper, iron, magnesium, manganese, molybdenum, phosphorus, selenium, zinc	A, B, C		
	Iron, magnesium, manganese, phosphorus, selenium, zinc	A, B, C, E		
	Copper, iron, manganese, zinc	B, K		
	Copper, iron, magnesium, manganese, molybdenum, phosphorus, selenium, zinc	A, B, C, E, K		

RANKING	FOOD	PROTEIN	FIBER	WHOLE GRAINS	HEALTHY FATS	
85	Scallops	✓			✓	
86	Green peas		✓			
87	Onions					
88	Chives		✓			
89	Garlic					
90	Whole-grain cereals		✓	✓	✓	
91	Dark chocolate					

CALCIUM	OTHER MINERALS	VITAMINS	POLYPHENOLS	FLAVONOIDS
	Copper, iron, magnesium, manganese, phosphorus, sodium, zinc	A, B, C, D, E		
	Copper, iodine, iron, magnesium, manganese, molybdenum, phosphorus, potassium, selenium, sodium, zinc	A, B, C, E, K		
	Chromium, copper, iodine, iron, magnesium, manganese, molybdenum, phosphorus, selenium, zinc	B, C, E, K	✓	
		A, B, C, K		
✓	Iron, selenium, manganese, copper, phosphorus	B, C		
	Iron	A, B		
	Magnesium, phosphorus, potassium	A	✓	

RANKING	FOOD	PROTEIN	FIBER	WHOLE GRAINS	HEALTHY FATS	
92	Flaxseed	✓	✓	✓	✓	
93	Pineapple		✓			
94	Corn		✓	✓		
95	Lean pork	✓				
96	Sunflower seeds	✓	✓			
97	Dried chile peppers					
98	Whey protein powder	✓				
99	Popcorn, air-popped, no butter		✓			
100	Vegetable juice, low-sodium					

CALCIUM	OTHER MINERALS	VITAMINS	POLYPHENOLS	FLAVONOIDS
	Copper, iron, magnesium, manganese, phosphorus, selenium, zinc	B, E		
	Copper, iron, magnesium, manganese, phosphorus, selenium, zinc	A, B, C, E, K		
	Copper, iron, magnesium, manganese, phosphorus, selenium, zinc	A, B, K		
	Iron, phosphorus, niacin			
	Copper, iron, magnesium, manganese, phosphorus, selenium, zinc	A, B, C, E, K		
	Potassium, iron	A, B, C		
	Potassium			
	Iron, manganese, phosphorus, magnesium			
	Iron	A, C		

Chapter 6

THE 20 WORST FOODS EVER
They're a Waste for Your Waist

EVERY SINGLE DAY, heinous crimes are committed against our bellies and our arteries. These nutritional crimes come in the form of misdemeanors (what's so bad about a candy bar now and then?) and felonies (daily bacon burgers). But some crimes are so bad, so egregious, and so gruesome that you'd hate to actually witness what goes on in your innards when these nutritional criminals are swallowed and allowed to wreak holy havoc on your body.

Now, you know my philosophy: One meal a week, it's okay to vacuum up your favorite foods as part of the ever-popular cheat meal. That will help you satisfy cravings so you're less likely to binge, gorge, and put buffets out of business the rest of the time. And I stick by it. That said, there are some food felons that are so evil they should be committed to death row, so that you never subject yourself to their malicious massacres of your waistline. Here are the 20 worst offenders. In the event you come face-to-face with one, don't try to fight it. Just get the hell away as fast as you can.

Worst Offender 1: Fettuccine Alfredo

Aliases: any pasta with (garlic/wine/tomato) cream sauce
Description: Often labeled as the world's worst food, just one serving of fettuccine Alfredo can top 1,000 calories and 90 grams of fat—a nutritional felon when the nonnutritious pasta made with bleached flour is topped with creamy and cheesy sauce. Better bet: whole-grain pasta topped with marinara or, for a heartier choice, tomato sauce with lean meat.

Worst Offender 2: Hardee's Monster Thickburger

Aliases: double burger, triple burger, and any "monster" or "big" burger
Description: At nearly 1,500 calories and 107 grams of fat, with ⅔ pound of beef, bacon, three slices of cheese, and mayo, this burger is considered extremely dangerous. While lean meat, including beef, is recommended for muscle building, the only thing this burger will build is your belly.

Worst Offender 3: Crème-Filled Doughnut with Chocolate Icing

Aliases: éclair, pastry, virtually any member of the doughnut family
Description: One Boston Kreme at Dunkin' Donuts has almost 250 calories and 9 grams of fat. Loaded with sugar, as well as saturated and trans fats, this breakfast bomb also causes collateral damage because it puts your blood sugar on a roller coaster, leaving you longing for more food very fast.

Worst Offender 4: Cinnabon Classic

Aliases: cinnamon roll, sweet roll, sticky bun
Description: This over-800-calorie "snack" or "dessert" packs 32 grams of fat and carries deadly weapons in the

form of diet-damaging sugar. However, it can be handled with caution, if you must tangle with one. Do damage control with a four-way split—enough to satisfy your sweet tooth, as well as your conscience.

Worst Offender 5: Deep-Fried Twinkies or Oreos

Aliases: deep-fried anything, especially at carnivals
Description: While a Twinkie itself contains a nutrient-free 150 calories and 5 grams of fat, deep-frying in oil nearly triples the calories. Fried Oreos? Over 100 calories *each* for that battered badness.

Worst Offender 6: Cheese Fries with Gravy

Alias: potato skins
Description: At more than 1,000 calories, this appetizer has a base of potatoes that's made with partially hydrogenated oil. Cheese and gravy smother the spuds with saturated fat.

Worst Offender 7: Soda

Aliases: Pop, cola, some high-cal energy drinks
Description: A 32-ounce Coke (which seems to be on the small side of serving cups these days) has more than 300 calories. If you guzzle high-cal drinks, switching to water and the occasional diet soda can immediately give you a huge caloric advantage. To wean yourself off the full-sugar stuff, start with a mixture that's three-quarters regular and a quarter diet. Every week, gradually change the ratio so that your tastebuds adjust to the difference in taste. Water down energy drinks so you retain some of the flavor (and electrolyte advantage if you work out a lot) without the extra calories.

Worst Offender 8: Bloomin' Onion

Aliases: onion loaf, fried onions, onion rings, any other fried "vegetable"

Description: It seems like a must to share one before a big steak dinner, but the deep-fried treatment turns a perfectly good vegetable into an insanely bad one. At more than 2,200 calories, this appetizer could fill your total daily caloric requirement.

Worst Offender 9: Spinach Dip and Chips or Bread

Aliases: most any fat-laden condiment

Description: Nothing wrong with the spinach. Nothing wrong with the artichokes. And nothing wrong with the fact that you're going to another Super Bowl party. But add in the other possible ingredients—sour cream, cream cheese, shredded cheese, and butter—and you're looking at a saturated-fat base sprinkled with some spinach. Add in refined flour in the form of bread or a 140 calories per 1-ounce serving of white corn chips, and you're scooping directly from mouth to gut.

Worst Offender 10: Pork Rinds

Alias: fried pig skin

Description: Just an ounce (about two handfuls) contains 150 calories, 10 grams of fat, and 500 milligrams of sodium. Often heralded by the no-carb crowd as a great snack with a savory bacon taste, the rinds are indeed great—for getting you closer to your first myocardial infarction. Plus, it's . . . fried . . . pig . . . skin.

Worst Offender 11: Potpie

Aliases: almost any full-fat frozen dinner

Description: With a crust made with heaps of butter and the gravy swimming in cream, these one-stop pies can top more than 500 calories per serving. Even though it's loaded with Powerfoods—chicken, turkey, vegetables—they're strangled by more than 30 grams of fat per serving.

Worst Offender 12: Sausage or Hot Dog

Aliases: bologna, pig in a blanket, bacon, any ultra-processed pork product

Description: Three dogs at the ballpark will cost you 900 calories, and that's not including the three beers to go with them. These nitrate-filled products go down fast—and that's why they're so dangerous. If you switch to turkey products, you can save yourself some serious fat and calories. A turkey dog, for instance, has half the calories of a beef one.

Worst Offender 13: Pizza Hut Stuffed-Crust Meat Lover's Pizza

Aliases: pizza with extra cheese, pepperoni, or sausage

Description: It's a double whammy: melted cheese and meat on top, as well as extra calories and fat stuffed inside the crust. One slice—*one slice!*—has 520 calories and 29 grams of fat. Next time you want to down half a pie, you're looking at more than 2,000 calories. Think of your stomach—that's what'll really be double stuffed.

Worst Offender 14: Cheesecake

Aliases: most restaurant desserts

Description: These huge hunks can have the caloric equivalent of an entire meal. Filled with, uh, cream cheese, this dessert tops 700 calories and leads to huge hunks on your hips.

Worst Offender 15: Movie-Theater Popcorn

Aliases: movie-theater nachos

Description: Nosh mindlessly while you watch Nicholson, De Niro, or Ferrell make movie history and you could eas-

ily take in 1,500 calories and more than 100 grams of fat
from the melted butter. Unfortunate, especially considering that butterless popcorn qualifies as a trusty whole
grain and serves as a perfect TV snack.

Worst Offender 16: Frosting

Aliases: glaze, icing
Description: As if the cake, doughnut, or cookie isn't filled
with enough sugar and white flour, its commercially prepared
frosting also contains trans fats (to keep it from melting), as
well as a truckload of sugar. A lick or two won't kill your
stomach; eating it by the spoonful just might.

Worst Offender 17: McDonald's Chocolate Triple Thick Shake

Aliases: many fast-food milkshakes and cream-filled coffee
drinks
Description: The McDonald's version holds 600 calories in
a 16-ounce cup, is high in fat and sugar, and contains high-
fructose corn syrup.

Worst Offender 18: Chicken Wings with Blue Cheese Dressing

Alias: fried chicken tenders
Description: Chicken—good. Chicken deep fried in vegetable
oil, coated with butter, and topped with a heavy-cream
dressing—bad. An order of 20 wings at Zaxby's, for instance,
tops 1,500 calories and nearly 100 grams of fat. And that's
without the blue cheese.

Worst Offender 19: Chips with Olestra

Aliases: chips with Olean
Description: In theory, it sounds great—a low-calorie
snack that contains an ingredient that prevents your body

from absorbing fat. But products made with olestra also deprive the body of vitamins that require fat for absorption, plus they have some ugly GI side effects. Blech.

Worst Offender 20: Your Calorie Kryptonite

Alias: the blob

Description: It might not appear on this list, but your nutritional worst nightmare is the food that you're always drawn to; the food you could eat and eat and eat; the food that tempts you every time you're stressed, sad, bored, or tired. And it's the food that will do you in every time. Ideally, you'll try to avoid it, but at the very least you can keep it under control if you can contain it to your cheat meal—so you satisfy your craving without fully giving in. That's why I really want you to take advantage of the weekly cheat meal. Indulge, enjoy, and long for the next time you'll have it. But if you try to ban your guiltiest pleasure forever, chances are that you simply won't—and that won't do any of us any good.

Chapter 7

POWERFOODS ANYWHERE, ANYTIME

A Complete Guide to Eating on the Run

USED TO BE that the only people who lived on the run were fugitives. These days, however, we're all running, all the time. Run to the store, to the bank, to school, to work, to kids' activities, to Mom's house to fix the sink, to the third-floor meeting, to the fifth-floor meeting, to check e-mail, to respond to e-mail, to the bathroom. It never ends. Our schedules never stop. And that means we're usually eating with one hand on the burger and the other on the cell phone or keyboard or steering wheel.

The ideal eating scenario involves taking a few minutes a day to decide what you're going to eat—and then taking a few more minutes to prepare it. That way, you have full control over what ingredients you use and, most important, how much you use. But I also know that there's about as much of a chance of you being able to consistently carve out that time as there is of Shaq giving Baryshnikov a run for his money.

I don't think that it's appropriate to admit defeat, however—no, not to the fast-food, grease-pit, pants-splitting establishments that have taken our collective belly hostage and threaten to kill us with each passing day. I understand that eating out and eating in the car are part of your life because of your work, family, and travel situations. So I want you to be prepared—prepared to make smart decisions, use your Powerfood rules no matter where you are, and enjoy eating out without sprouting out.

Below, to make things easier, I've listed the smartest (and worst) choices at some popular fast-food and chain restaurants, as well as some generic places, so you can make good decisions no matter where you eat. (For the record, some popular chains like Outback, Olive Garden, T.G.I. Fridays, and Hooters do not release their nutritional information to the public and did not respond to our requests for it.) These choices are based not only on total calories or saturated fat but also on the complete picture of balancing out important nutrients.

Arby's

Best Meals

Ham & Swiss Melt Sandwich and Martha's Vineyard Salad: 552 calories, 44 g protein, 59 g carbohydrates, 14 g total fat, 6 g saturated fat, 0 g trans fat, 99 mg cholesterol, 6 g fiber, 1,572 mg sodium, 23 g sugar

Santa Fe Salad with Grilled Chicken: 305 calories, 30 g protein, 21 g carbohydrates, 11 g total fat, 6 g saturated fat, 0 g trans fat, 78 mg cholesterol, 6 g fiber, 621 mg sodium, 8 g sugar

Worst Choice

Ultimate BLT Sandwich: 779 calories, 23 g protein, 75 g carbohydrates, 45 g total fat, 11 g saturated fat, 1 g trans fat, 51 mg cholesterol, 6 g fiber, 1,571 mg sodium, 18 g sugar

Choice That Sounds Good for You but Isn't

Chicken Salad with Pecans Wrap: 638 calories, 30 g protein, 48 g carbohydrates, 38 g total fat, 10 g saturated fat, 0 g trans fat, 74 mg cholesterol, 8 g fiber, 1,199 mg sodium, 3 g sugar

Atlanta Bread Company

Best Meals

Chopstix Chicken Salad with Fat-Free Raspberry Vinaigrette: 315 calories, 19 g protein, 32 g carbohydrates, 13 g total fat, 1.5 g saturated fat, n/a g trans fat, 40 mg cholesterol, 5 g fiber, 780 mg sodium, 16 g sugar

Roasted Turkey Breast on Nine Grain Bread: 430 calories, 32 g protein, 61 g carbohydrates, 7 g total fat, 2 g saturated fat, n/a g trans fat, 35 mg cholesterol, 5 g fiber, 1,350 mg sodium, 8 g sugar

Tangy Roast Beef Sandwich and Garden Vegetable Soup: 490 calories, 35 g protein, 75 g carbohydrates, 5.5 g total fat, 2.5 g saturated fat, n/a g trans fat, 50 mg cholesterol, 7 g fiber, 2,190 mg sodium, 7 g sugar

Worst Choice

Basil Pesto Pasta: 940 calories, 46 g protein, 69 g carbohydrates, 53 g total fat, 10 g saturated fat, n/a g trans fat, 120 mg cholesterol, 4 g fiber, 1,510 mg sodium, 8 g sugar

Choice That Sounds Good for You but Isn't

California Avocado on Tomato Onion Focaccia: 690 calories, 14 g protein, 71 g carbohydrates, 40 g total fat, 7 g saturated fat, n/a g trans fat, 15 mg cholesterol, 14 g fiber, 1,010 mg sodium, 10 g sugar

Baja Fresh

Best Meals

Bare Chicken Burrito (Served in a Bowl): 640 calories, 45 g protein, 97 g carbohydrates, 7 g total fat, 1 g saturated fat, 0 g trans fat, 75 mg cholesterol, 20 g fiber, 2,330 mg sodium, n/a g sugar

Carnitas Baja Taco and Side Salad with Fat Free Salsa Verde: 365 calories, 15 g protein, 48 g carbohydrates, 13 g total fat, 3.5 g saturated fat, 0 g trans fat, 25 mg cholesterol, 7 g fiber, 1,080 mg sodium, n/a g sugar

Worst Choice

Steak Nachos: 2,120 calories, 96 g protein, 163 g carbohydrates, 118 g total fat, 44 g saturated fat, 4.5 g trans fat, 255 mg cholesterol, 31 g fiber, 2,990 mg sodium, n/a g sugar

Choice That Sounds Good for You but Isn't

Chipotle Glazed Steak Salad: 700 calories, 54 g protein, 54 g carbohydrates, 31 g total fat, 11 g saturated fat, 2 g trans fat, 135 mg cholesterol, 9 g fiber, 1,140 mg sodium, n/a g sugar

Boston Market

Best Meals

Roasted Turkey with Broccoli in Garlic Butter and Green Beans: 320 calories, 43 g protein, 13 g carbohydrates, 12.5 g total fat, 4.5 g saturated fat, 0 g trans fat, 70 mg cholesterol, 6 g fiber, 1,030 mg sodium, 3 g sugar

¼ White Rotisserie Chicken (skinless), Garlic Dill New Potatoes, and Fresh Steamed Vegetables: 410 calories, 47 g protein, 38 g carbohydrates, 7 g total fat, 1.5 g saturated fat, 0 g trans fat, 135 mg cholesterol, 6 g fiber, 800 mg sodium, 5 g sugar

Worst Choice

Boston Meatloaf Carver: 940 calories, 49 g protein, 96 g carbohydrates, 45 g total fat, 18 g saturated fat, 0 g trans fat, 155 mg cholesterol, 6 g fiber, 2,080 mg sodium, 11 g sugar

Choice That Sounds Good for You but Isn't

Market Chopped Side Salad: 440 calories, 4 g protein, 12 g carbohydrates, 43 g total fat, 7 g saturated fat, 1 g trans fat, 5 mg cholesterol, 3 g fiber, 1,790 mg sodium, 7 g sugar

Burger King

Best Meals

Whopper Jr. Sandwich without mayo and Garden Salad (no chicken) with Ken's Fat Free Ranch Dressing: 440 calories,

20 g protein, 53 g carbohydrates, 17 g total fat, 7 g saturated fat, 0 g trans fat, 55 mg cholesterol, 7 g fiber, 1,355 mg sodium, 14 g sugar

Tendergrill Chicken Garden Salad with Ken's Light Italian Dressing: 360 calories, 33 g protein, 13 g carbohydrates, 20 g total fat, 5 g saturated fat, 0 g trans fat, 80 mg cholesterol, 4 g fiber, 1,160 mg sodium, 7 g sugar

Worst Choice

Triple Whopper Sandwich with Cheese and Mayo: 1,230 calories, 71 g protein, 52 g carbohydrates, 82 g total fat, 32 g saturated fat, 3.5 g trans fat, 275 mg cholesterol, 3 g fiber, 1,590 mg sodium, 11 g sugar

Choice That Sounds Good for You but Isn't

BK Fish Filet Sandwich with Tartar Sauce: 630 calories, 24 g protein, 67 g carbohydrates, 30 g total fat, 6 g saturated fat, 2.5 g trans fat, 60 mg cholesterol, 4 g fiber, 1,380 mg sodium, 8 g sugar

Chick-fil-A

Best Meals

Chargrilled Chicken Cool Wrap and Carrot & Raisin Salad: 580 calories, 35 g protein, 74 g carbohydrates, 18 g total fat, 4.5 g saturated fat, 0 g trans fat, 80 mg cholesterol, 10 g fiber, 1,420 mg sodium, 25 g sugar

Chick-fil-A Southwest Chargrilled Salad with Reduced Fat Raspberry Vinaigrette and Fruit Cup: 390 calories, 26 g protein, 48 g carbohydrates, 10 g total fat, 3.5 g saturated fat, 0 g trans fat, 60 mg cholesterol, 7 g fiber, 960 mg sodium, 30 g sugar

Chick-fil-A Chargrilled Chicken Sandwich and Side Salad with Light Italian Dressing: 345 calories, 31 g protein, 39 g carbohydrates, 7 g total fat, 2.5 g saturated fat, 0 g trans fat, 75 mg cholesterol, 5 g fiber, 1,585 mg sodium, 11 g sugar

Worst Choice

Chicken Deluxe Sandwich: 420 calories, 28 g protein, 39 g carbohydrates, 16 g total fat, 3.5 g saturated fat, 0 g trans fat, 60 mg cholesterol, 2 g fiber, 1,300 mg sodium, 5 g sugar

Choice That Sounds Good for You but Isn't

Chick-fil-A Chick-n-Strips Salad: 400 calories, 34 g protein, 21 g carbohydrates, 20 g total fat, 6 g saturated fat, 0 g trans fat, 80 mg cholesterol, 4 g fiber, 1,070 mg sodium, 7 g sugar

Chili's

Best Meals

Guiltless Black Bean Burger on a Whole Wheat Bun (Unbuttered) and a House Dinner Salad with Non-Fat Honey Mustard Dressing: 520 calories, 57 g protein, 38 g carbohydrates, 12 g total fat, 3 g saturated fat, n/a g trans fat, n/a mg cholesterol, 24 g fiber, 1,170 mg sodium, n/a g sugar

Guiltless Salmon and Seasonal Veggies: 570 calories, 58 g protein, 39 g carbohydrates, 20 g total fat, 4 g saturated fat, n/a g trans fat, n/a mg cholesterol, 13 g fiber, 1,190 mg sodium, n/a g sugar

Guiltless Chicken Platter and cup of Southwestern Vegetable Soup: 690 calories, 44 g protein, 98 g carbohydrates, 14 g total fat, 5 g saturated fat, n/a g trans fat, n/a mg cholesterol, 7 g fiber, 3,400 mg sodium, n/a g sugar

Worst Choice

Fajita Steak Quesadillas with Guacamole: 2,030 calories, 102 g protein, 150 g carbohydrates, 111 g total fat, 53 g saturated fat, n/a g trans fat, n/a mg cholesterol, 17 g fiber, 5,680 mg sodium, n/a g sugar

Choice That Sounds Good for You but Isn't

Steak & Portobello Fajitas: 1,130 calories, 65 g protein, 26 g carbohydrates, 84 g total fat, 22 g saturated fat, n/a g trans fat, n/a mg cholesterol, 5 g fiber, 3,850 mg sodium, n/a g sugar

Domino's

Best Meals

12-inch Medium One-Topping Crunchy Thin Crust Pizza (1 slice): 130 calories, 5 g protein, 14 g carbohydrates, 8.5 g total fat, 2.5 g saturated fat, 0 g trans fat, 10 mg cholesterol, 1 g fiber, 240 mg sodium, 2 g sugar

Grilled Chicken Caesar Salad with Creamy Caesar Dressing: 315 calories, 13 g protein, 8 g carbohydrates, 26 g total fat, 5.5 g saturated fat, 0 g trans fat, 35 mg cholesterol, 1 g fiber, 830 mg sodium, 4 g sugar

12-inch Medium Crunchy Thin Crust Vegi Feast Pizza (1 slice): 160 calories, 7 g protein, 16 g carbohydrates, 9.5 g total fat, 3.5 g saturated fat, 0 g trans fat, 15 mg cholesterol, 2 g fiber, 355 mg sodium, 2 g sugar

Worst Choice

14-inch Large Ultimate Deep Dish MeatZZa Feast (1 slice): 440 calories, 18 g protein, 42 g carbohydrates, 24 g total fat, 9.5 g saturated fat, 0 g trans fat, 40 mg cholesterol, 5 g fiber, 1,160 mg sodium, 2 g sugar

Choice That Sounds Good for You but Isn't

12-inch medium Classic Hand Tossed with Grilled Chicken (1 slice): 230 calories, 12 g protein, 30 g carbohydrates, 8 g total fat, 3 g saturated fat, 0 g trans fat, 20 mg cholesterol, 1 g fiber, 425 mg sodium, 4 g sugar

Don Pablo's

Best Meals

Mamma's Skinny Enchiladas (3) without rice or garnish and Pecos Valley Vegetables: 466 calories, 27 g protein, 31 g carbohydrates, 19 g total fat, 6 g saturated fat, n/a g trans fat, 73 mg cholesterol, 7 g fiber, 2,333 mg sodium, 10 g sugar

Grilled Chicken Parrilla with Black Beans: 660 calories, 53 g protein, 79 g carbohydrates, 11 g total fat, 2 g saturated fat, n/a g trans fat, 122 mg cholesterol, 14 g fiber, 2,544 mg sodium, 18 g sugar

Worst Choice

Spicy Taco Meat Nachos: 1,625 calories, 70 g protein, 85 g carbohydrates, 113 g total fat, 55 g saturated fat, n/a g trans fat, 242 mg cholesterol, 14 g fiber, 3,308 mg sodium, 22 g sugar

Choice That Sounds Good for You but Isn't

Steak Caesar Salad: 1,792 calories, 37 g protein, 97 g carbohydrates, 144 g total fat, 31 g saturated fat, n/a g trans fat, 119 mg cholesterol, 11 g fiber, 2,886 mg sodium, 38 g sugar

Dunkin' Donuts

Best Meals

Reduced Carb Bagel with Cheese: 380 calories, 25 g protein, 45 g carbohydrates, 12 g total fat, 4.5 g saturated fat, 0 g trans fat, 20 mg cholesterol, 14 g fiber, 780 mg sodium, 8 g sugar

Egg Cheese English Muffin Sandwich: 280 calories, 15 g protein, 34 g carbohydrates, 9 g total fat, 4.5 g saturated fat, 0 g trans fat, 140 mg cholesterol, 1 g fiber, 1,010 mg sodium, 3 g sugar

Small Mango Passion Fruits Smoothie: 360 calories, 7 g protein, 79 g carbohydrates, 2.5 g total fat, 1.5 g saturated fat, 0 g trans fat, 10 mg cholesterol, 2 g fiber, 120 mg sodium, 68 g sugar

Worst Choice

Sausage Egg Cheese Croissant Sandwich: 690 calories, 22 g protein, 40 g carbohydrates, 51 g total fat, 17 g saturated fat, 7 g trans fat, 230 mg cholesterol, 0 g fiber, 1,080 mg sodium, 8 g sugar

Choice That Sounds Good for You but Isn't

Plain Cake Munchkins (4): 270 calories, 3 g protein, 27 g carbohydrates, 16 g total fat, 4 g saturated fat, 4 g trans fat, 25 mg cholesterol, 1 g fiber, 240 mg sodium, 9 g sugar

Multigrain Bagel with Plain Cream Cheese: 570 calories, 18 g protein, 72 g carbohydrates, 23 g total fat, 14 g saturated fat, 0 g trans fat, 55 mg cholesterol, 5 g fiber, 840 mg sodium, 9 g sugar

Hardee's

Best Meals

Regular Roast Beef Sandwich and Small Mashed Potatoes: 420 calories, 20 g protein, 46 g carbohydrates, 18 g total fat, 7 g saturated fat, n/a g trans fat, 40 mg cholesterol, 2 g fiber, 1,270 mg sodium, 3 g sugar

Charbroiled BBQ Chicken Sandwich and Small Cole Slaw: 585 calories, 37 g protein, 78 g carbohydrates, 15 g total fat, 3 g saturated fat, n/a g trans fat, 70 mg cholesterol, 6 g fiber, 1,315 mg sodium, 29 g sugar

Worst Choice

Monster Thickburger: 1,410 calories, 60 g protein, 47 g carbohydrates, 107 g total fat, 45 g saturated fat, n/a g trans fat, 229 mg cholesterol, 2 g fiber, 2,740 mg sodium, 9 g sugar

Choice That Sounds Good for You but Isn't

1/3-Lb. Low Carb Thickburger: 420 calories, 30 g protein, 5 g carbohydrates, 32 g total fat, 12 g saturated fat, n/a g trans fat, 115 mg cholesterol, 2 g fiber, 1,010 mg sodium, 3 g sugar

Kentucky Fried Chicken

Best Meals

Tender Roast Sandwich (without sauce) and Green Beans: 350 calories, 39 g protein, 35 g carbohydrates, 6 g total fat, 1.5 g saturated fat, 0 g trans fat, 75 mg cholesterol, 4 g fiber, 1,630 mg sodium, 5 g sugar

Roasted Caesar Salad (without croutons) with Hidden Valley Golden Italian Light Dressing and Corn on the Cob (3-inch): 330 calories, 32 g protein, 25 g carbohydrates, 12 g total fat, 5 g saturated fat, 0 g trans fat, 70 mg cholesterol, 6 g fiber, 1,490 mg sodium, 13 g sugar

Worst Choice

KFC Famous Mashed Potato Bowl with Gravy: 740 calories, 27 g protein, 80 g carbohydrates, 35 g total fat, 9 g saturated fat, 1.5 g trans fat, 60 mg cholesterol, 7 g fiber, 2,350 mg sodium, 6 g sugar

Choice That Sounds Good for You but Isn't

Crispy Caesar Salad (without dressing or croutons): 350 calories, 29 g protein, 16 g carbohydrates, 19 g total fat, 6 g saturated fat, 0 g trans fat, 70 mg cholesterol, 3 g fiber, 1,080 mg sodium, 3 g sugar

McDonald's

Best Meals

Asian Salad with Grilled Chicken with Newman's Own Low Fat Balsamic Vinaigrette: 340 calories, 32 g protein, 27 g carbohydrates, 12 g total fat, 1.5 g saturated fat, 0 g trans fat, 65 mg cholesterol, 5 g fiber, 1,620 mg sodium, 16 g sugar

Premium Grilled Chicken Classic Sandwich and Side Salad with Newman's Own Low Fat Balsamic Vinaigrette: 480 calories, 33 g protein, 58 g carbohydrates, 13 g total fat, 2.5 g saturated fat, 0 g trans fat, 70 mg cholesterol, 5 g fiber, 1,930 mg sodium, 16 g sugar

Hamburger and Asian Salad (without chicken) with Newman's Own Low Fat Family Recipe Italian Dressing: 460 calories, 21 g protein, 55 g carbohydrates, 18 g total fat, 4 g saturated fat, 0.5 g trans fat, 30 mg cholesterol, 7 g fiber, 1,280 mg sodium, 16 g sugar

Worst Choice

Chicken McNuggets (20 pieces): 840 calories, 50 g protein, 51 g carbohydrates, 49 g total fat, 11 g saturated fat, 5 g trans fat, 125 mg cholesterol, 0 g fiber, 2,240 mg sodium, 0 g sugar

Choice That Sounds Good for You but Isn't

Chicken Select Premium Breast Strips (5 pieces): 630 calories, 39 g protein, 46 g carbohydrates, 33 g total fat, 6 g saturated fat, 4.5 g trans fat, 90 mg cholesterol, 0 g fiber, 1,550 mg sodium, 0 g sugar

Panda Express

Best Meals

Mushroom Chicken with Steamed Rice and Mixed Vegetables: 600 calories, 22 g protein, 96 g carbohydrates, 15.5 g total fat, 3 g saturated fat, 0 g trans fat, 45 mg cholesterol, 10 g fiber, 660 mg sodium, 7 g sugar

Broccoli Beef with Steamed Rice: 530 calories, 20 g protein, 92 g carbohydrates, 9.5 g total fat, 2 g saturated fat, 0 g trans fat, 25 mg cholesterol, 8 g fiber, 540 mg sodium, 3 g sugar

Worst Choice

Orange Chicken: 500 calories, 23 g protein, 42 g carbohydrates, 27 g total fat, 5.5 g saturated fat, 1 g trans fat, 100 mg cholesterol, 3 g fiber, 810 mg sodium, 14 g sugar

Choice That Sounds Good for You but Isn't

Mandarin Chicken: 250 calories, 31 g protein, 8 g carbohydrates, 10 g total fat, 3 g saturated fat, 0 g trans fat, 145 mg cholesterol, 0 g fiber, 1,150 mg sodium, 8 g sugar

Panera Bread

Best Meals

Tomato & Fresh Basil Crispani and Fresh Fruit Cup (10 oz): 470 calories, 15 g protein, 74 g carbohydrates, 13 g total fat, 6 g saturated fat, 0 g trans fat, 20 mg cholesterol, 4 g fiber, 580 mg sodium, 24 g sugar

Asian Sesame Chicken Salad with fat-free raspberry dressing: 500 calories, 33 g protein, 42 g carbohydrates, 22 g total fat, 3 g saturated fat, 0 g trans fat, 65 mg cholesterol, 6 g fiber, 1,125 mg sodium, 17 g sugar

Lowfat Chicken Noodle Soup: 100 calories, 5 g protein, 15 g carbohydrates, 2 g total fat, 0 g saturated fat, 0 g trans fat, 15 mg cholesterol, 1 g fiber, 1,080 mg sodium, 1 g sugar

Worst Choice

Italian Combo Signature Sandwich: 1,110 calories, 61 g protein, 91 g carbohydrates, 56 g total fat, 20 g saturated fat, 0 g trans fat, 180 mg cholesterol, 5 g fiber, 3,220 mg sodium, 5 g sugar

Choice That Sounds Good for You but Isn't

Bistro Steak Hand-Tossed Salad: 630 calories, 22 g protein, 16 g carbohydrates, 57 g total fat, 12 g saturated fat, 0 g trans fat, 55 mg cholesterol, 4 g fiber, 940 mg sodium, 8 g sugar

Papa John's

Best Meals

12-inch Garden Fresh Original Crust Pizza (1 slice): 200 calories, 8 g protein, 28 g carbohydrates, 7 g total fat, 2 g saturated fat, 0 g trans fat, 10 mg cholesterol, 2 g fiber, 490 mg sodium, 4 g sugar

12-inch Original Crust Cheese Pizza (1 slice): 210 calories, 9 g protein, 27 g carbohydrates, 8 g total fat, 2.5 g saturated fat, 0 g trans fat, 15 mg cholesterol, 1 g fiber, 510 mg sodium, 3 g sugar

Worst Choice

12-inch Sausage Sensation Pan Crust Pizza (1 slice): 440 calories, 15 g protein, 41 g carbohydrates, 22 g total fat, 10 g saturated fat, 0 g trans fat, 30 mg cholesterol, 2 g fiber, 1,070 mg sodium, 5 g sugar

Choice That Sounds Good for You but Isn't

14-inch Thin Crust Cheese Pizza (1 slice): 240 calories, 10 g protein, 22 g carbohydrates, 13 g total fat, 3.5 g saturated fat, 0 g trans fat, 20 mg cholesterol, 1 g fiber, 500 mg sodium, 2 g sugar

P.F. Chang's China Bistro

Best Meals

Ginger Chicken & Broccoli: 660 calories, 61 g protein, 45 g carbohydrates, 26 g total fat, 3.5 g saturated fat, n/a g trans fat, n/a mg cholesterol, n/a g fiber, n/a mg sodium, n/a g sugar

Oolong Marinated Sea Bass: 520 calories, 63 g protein, 40 g carbohydrates, 12 g total fat, 2.5 g saturated fat, n/a g trans fat, n/a mg cholesterol, n/a g fiber, n/a mg sodium, n/a g sugar

Worst Choice

Lo Mein Pork (for dinner): 1,820 calories, 63 g protein, 95 g carbohydrates, 127 g total fat, 23 g saturated fat, n/a g trans fat, n/a mg cholesterol, n/a g fiber, n/a mg sodium, n/a g sugar

Choice That Sounds Good for You but Isn't

Philip's Better Lemon Chicken: 1,060 calories, 58 g protein, 113 g carbohydrates, 42 g total fat, 6 g saturated fat, n/a g trans fat, n/a mg cholesterol, n/a g fiber, n/a mg sodium, n/a g sugar

Pizza Hut

Best Meals

12-inch Medium Quartered Ham and Pineapple Thin 'N Crispy Pizza (1 slice): 180 calories, 9 g protein, 23 g carbohydrates, 6 g total fat, 3 g saturated fat, 0 g trans fat, 20 mg cholesterol, 1 g fiber, 570 mg sodium, 4 g sugar

12-inch Fit 'N Delicious Green Pepper, Red Onion & Diced Red Tomato Pizza (1 slice): 150 calories, 6 g protein, 23 g carbohydrates, 4 g total fat, 1.5 g saturated fat, 0 g trans fat, 10 mg cholesterol, 1 g fiber, 420 mg sodium, 4 g sugar

12-inch Fit 'N Delicious Diced Red Tomato, Mushroom, and Jalapeño Pizza (1 slice): 150 calories, 6 g protein, 22 g carbohydrates, 4 g total fat, 1.5 g saturated fat, 0 g trans fat, 10 mg cholesterol, 1 g fiber, 630 mg sodium, 4 g sugar

Worst Choice

14-inch large Meat Lover's Pan Pizza (1 slice): 530 calories, 23 g protein, 39 g carbohydrates, 31 g total fat, 11 g saturated fat, 0.5 g trans fat, 65 mg cholesterol, 2 g fiber, 1,400 mg sodium, 3 g sugar

Choice That Sounds Good for You but Isn't

6-inch Personal Pan Cheese Pizza: 620 calories, 28 g protein, 69 g carbohydrates, 26 g total fat, 11 g saturated fat, 0.5 g trans fat, 60 mg cholesterol, 3 g fiber, 1,370 mg sodium, 7 g sugar

Romano's Macaroni Grill

Best Meals

Simple Salmon: 590 calories, 47 g protein, 5 g carbohydrates, 40 g total fat, 6 g saturated fat, n/a g trans fat, n/a mg cholesterol, 2 g fiber, 1,390 mg sodium, n/a g sugar

Pollo Magra "Skinny Chicken" and cup of Italian Sausage and Tomato Soup: 520 calories, 50 g protein, 51 g carbohydrates, 12 g total fat, 3 g saturated fat, n/a g trans fat, n/a mg cholesterol, 8 g fiber, 1,720 mg sodium, n/a g sugar

Worst Choice

Spaghetti & Meatballs with meat sauce (dinner): 2,430 calories, 96 g protein, 207 g carbohydrates, 128 g total fat, 57 g saturated fat, n/a g trans fat, n/a mg cholesterol, 14 g fiber, 5,290 mg sodium, n/a g sugar

Choice That Sounds Good for You but Isn't

Grilled Salmon with Honey-Teriyaki Glaze: 1,230 calories, 56 g protein, 79 g carbohydrates, 74 g total fat, 9 g saturated fat, n/a g trans fat, n/a mg cholesterol, 5 g fiber, 6,590 mg sodium, n/a g sugar

Ruby Tuesday

Best Meals

Top Sirloin with Premium Baby Green Beans and Garden Vegetable Soup: 524 calories, n/a g protein, 25 g carbohydrates, 18 g total fat, n/a g saturated fat, n/a g trans fat, n/a mg cholesterol, 6 g fiber, n/a mg sodium, n/a g sugar

Creole Catch: 662 calories, n/a g protein, 38 g carbohydrates, 31 g total fat, n/a g saturated fat, n/a g trans fat, n/a mg cholesterol, 5 g fiber, n/a mg sodium, n/a g sugar

Worst Choice

Colossal Burger: 1,943 calories, n/a g protein, 74 g carbohydrates, 141 g total fat, n/a g saturated fat, n/a g trans fat, n/a mg cholesterol, 7 g fiber, n/a mg sodium, n/a g sugar

Choice That Sounds Good for You but Isn't

Fresh Chicken & Broccoli Pasta: 2,061 calories, n/a g protein, 109 g carbohydrates, 128 g total fat, n/a g saturated fat, n/a g trans fat, n/a mg cholesterol, 13 g fiber, n/a mg sodium, n/a g sugar

Sbarro

Best Meals

Low Carb Cheese Pizza Slice: 310 calories, 34 g protein, 18 g carbohydrates, 14 g total fat, n/a g saturated fat, n/a g trans fat, 25 mg cholesterol, 0 g fiber, 640 mg sodium, n/a g sugar

Meatballs and a Pasta Primavera Salad: 330 calories, 12 g protein, 31 g carbohydrates, 19 g total fat, n/a g saturated fat, n/a g trans fat, 30 mg cholesterol, 3 g fiber, 2,060 mg sodium, n/a g sugar

Worst Choice

Stuffed Pepperoni Pizza Slice: 960 calories, 52 g protein, 89 g carbohydrates, 42 g total fat, n/a g saturated fat, n/a g trans fat, 115 mg cholesterol, 4 g fiber, 3,200 mg sodium, n/a g sugar

Choice That Sounds Good for You but Isn't

Chicken Portofino: 730 calories, 63 g protein, 7 g carbohydrates, 48 g total fat, n/a g saturated fat, n/a g trans fat, 225 mg cholesterol, 1 g fiber, 790 mg sodium, n/a g sugar

Schlotzsky's

Best Meals

Mediterranean Tuna Wrap: 324 calories, 19 g protein, 48 g carbohydrates, 7 g total fat, n/a g saturated fat, 0 g trans fat, 33 mg cholesterol, 5 g fiber, 1,124 mg sodium, n/a g sugar

Cup of Hearty Vegetable Beef Soup and Grilled Chicken Caesar Salad: 330 calories, 59 g protein, 24 g carbohydrates, 13 g total fat, n/a g saturated fat, 0 g trans fat, 80 mg cholesterol, 5 g fiber, 1,779 mg sodium, n/a g sugar

Medium Smoked Turkey Breast Oven-Toasted Sandwich: 500 calories, 33 g protein, 76 g carbohydrates, 7 g total fat, n/a g saturated fat, 0 g trans fat, 59 mg cholesterol, 4 g fiber, 1,806 mg sodium, n/a g sugar

Worst Choice

Medium Turkey Original-Style Oven-Toasted Sandwich: 815 calories, 51 g protein, 78 g carbohydrates, 33 g total fat, n/a g saturated fat, 1 g trans fat, 132 mg cholesterol, 4 g fiber, 2,770 mg sodium, n/a g sugar

Choice That Sounds Good for You but Isn't

Parmesan Chicken Caesar Salad Wrap: 514 calories, 52 g protein, 47 g carbohydrates, 26 g total fat, n/a g saturated fat, 0 g trans fat, 68 mg cholesterol, 5 g fiber, 1,440 mg sodium, n/a g sugar

Starbucks

Best Meals

Lowfat Blueberry Muffin: 270 calories, 5 g protein, 58 g carbohydrates, 2 g total fat, 0.5 g saturated fat, 0 g trans fat, 55 mg cholesterol, 2 g fiber, 650 mg sodium, 28 g sugar

Reduced-Fat Blueberry Coffee Cake: 310 calories, 4 g protein, 58 g carbohydrates, 10 g total fat, 6 g saturated fat, 0 g trans fat, 10 mg cholesterol, 1 g fiber, 420 mg sodium, 35 g sugar

Worst Choice

Chocolate Chunk Cookie: 460 calories, 7 g protein, 56 g carbohydrates, 27 g total fat, 17 g saturated fat, 0 g trans fat, 40 mg cholesterol, 5 g fiber, 410 mg sodium, 24 g sugar

Choice That Sounds Good for You but Isn't

Oat, Fruit and Nut Cookie: 370 calories, 6 g protein, 49 g carbohydrates, 18 g total fat, 7 g saturated fat, 0 g trans fat, 55 mg cholesterol, 3 g fiber, 480 mg sodium, 29 g sugar

Banana Nut Loaf: 460 calories, 7 g protein, 56 g carbohydrates, 24 g total fat, 10 g saturated fat, 0 g trans fat, 105 mg cholesterol, 2 g fiber, 360 mg sodium, 32 g sugar

Subway

Best Meals

6-inch Turkey Breast and Ham on Wheat: 290 calories, 20 g protein, 47 g carbohydrates, 5 g total fat, 1.5 g saturated fat, 0 g trans fat, 25 mg cholesterol, 4 g fiber, 1,210 mg sodium, 8 g sugar

6-inch Oven Roasted Chicken Breast: 310 calories, 24 g protein, 48 g carbohydrates, 5 g total fat, 1.5 g saturated fat, 0 g trans fat, 25 mg cholesterol, 5 g fiber, 830 mg sodium, 9 g sugar

Turkey Breast Wrap and Minestrone: 350 calories, 20 g protein, 54 g carbohydrates, 7 g total fat, 2 g saturated fat, 0 g trans fat, 25 mg cholesterol, 7 g fiber, 2,235 mg sodium, 8 g sugar

Worst Choice

6-inch Meatball Marinara: 560 calories, 24 g protein, 63 g carbohydrates, 24 g total fat, 11 g saturated fat, 1 g trans fat, 45 mg cholesterol, 7 g fiber, 1,590 mg sodium, 13 g sugar

Choice That Sounds Good for You but Isn't

6" Tuna: 530 calories, 22 g protein, 44 g carbohydrates, 31 g total fat, 76 g saturated fat, 0.5 g trans fat, 45 mg cholesterol, 4 g fiber, 1,010 mg sodium, 7 g sugar

Taco Bell

Best Meals

Chicken Gorditas Baja without cheese or sauce (2): 460 calories, 30 g protein, 54 g carbohydrates, 14 g total fat, 3 g saturated fat, 0 g trans fat, 50 mg cholesterol, 5 g fiber, 1,270 mg sodium, 10 g sugar

Chicken Burrito Supreme without cheese or sauce: 360 calories, 18 g protein, 47 g carbohydrates, 11 g total fat, 4.5 g saturated fat, 0.5 g trans fat, 35 mg cholesterol, 6 g fiber, 1,080 mg sodium, 5 g sugar

Grilled Steak Soft Tacos (2): 320 calories, 20 g protein, 40 g carbohydrates, 9 g total fat, 3.5 g saturated fat, 0 g trans fat, 35 mg cholesterol, 4 g fiber, 1,110 mg sodium, 5 g sugar

Worst Choice

Fiesta Taco Salad: 840 calories, 30 g protein, 80 g carbohydrates, 45 g total fat, 11 g saturated fat, 1.5 g trans fat, 65 mg cholesterol, 15 g fiber, 1,780 mg sodium, 10 g sugar

Choice That Sounds Good for You but Isn't:

Grilled Chicken Stuft Burrito: 640 calories, 34 g protein, 73 g carbohydrates, 23 g total fat, 7 g saturated fat, 0.5 g trans fat, 65 mg cholesterol, 7 g fiber, 2,160 mg sodium, 6 g sugar

Wendy's

Best Meals

Large Chili and Side Salad with Fat Free French Style Dressing: 440 calories, 27 g protein, 62 g carbohydrates, 10 g total fat, 3.5 g saturated fat, 0.5 g trans fat, 55 mg cholesterol, 11 g fiber, 1,410 mg sodium, 29 g sugar

Roasted Turkey & Basil Pesto Frescata and Mandarin Oranges: 500 calories, 22 g protein, 69 g carbohydrates, 15 g total fat, 3 g saturated fat, 0 g trans fat, 40 mg cholesterol, 5 g fiber, 1,535 mg sodium, 20 g sugar

Worst Choice

Big Bacon Classic: 590 calories, 34 g protein, 46 g carbohydrates, 30 g total fat, 12 g saturated fat, 1.5 g trans fat, 90 mg cholesterol, 3 g fiber, 1,510 mg sodium, 11 g sugar

Choice That Sounds Good for You but Isn't:

Southwest Taco Salad: 710 calories, 34 g protein, 51 g carbohydrates, 41 g total fat, 17 g saturated fat, 1.5 g trans fat, 105 mg cholesterol, 10 g fiber, 1,620 mg sodium, 14 g sugar

Your Favorite Chinese Restaurant

Best Meals

Shrimp with Lobster Sauce: 480 calories, 42 g protein, 24 g carbohydrates, 22 g total fat, 3.5 g saturated fat, n/a g trans fat, n/a mg cholesterol, n/a g fiber, n/a mg sodium, n/a g sugar

Moo Goo Gai Pan: 660 calories, 54 g protein, 32 g carbohydrates, 34 g total fat, 3.5 g saturated fat, n/a g trans fat, n/a mg cholesterol, n/a g fiber, n/a mg sodium, n/a g sugar

Worst Choice

Lo Mein Combo: 1,820 calories, 66 g protein, 98 g carbohydrates, 126 g total fat, 20 g saturated fat, n/a g trans fat, n/a mg cholesterol, n/a g fiber, n/a mg sodium, n/a g sugar

Choice That Sounds Good for You but Isn't

Beef with Broccoli: 1,120 calories, 93 g protein, 38 g carbohydrates, 65 g total fat, 16 g saturated fat, n/a g trans fat, n/a mg cholesterol, n/a g fiber, n/a mg sodium, n/a g sugar

Your Favorite Italian Restaurant

Best Meals

Bowl of Pasta e Fagioli Soup: 760 calories, 28 g protein, 88 g carbohydrates, 31 g total fat, 5 g saturated fat, n/a g trans fat, n/a mg cholesterol, 21 g fiber, 1,980 mg sodium, n/a g sugar

Sausage and Peppers with Pasta: 860 calories, 29 g protein, 84 g carbohydrates, 45 g total fat, 24 g saturated fat, n/a g trans fat, n/a mg cholesterol, 9 g fiber, 2,470 mg sodium, n/a g sugar

Worst Choice

Fettuccine Alfredo with Chicken: 1,370 calories, 51 g protein, 68 g carbohydrates, 97 g total fat, 56 g saturated fat, n/a g trans fat, n/a mg cholesterol, 4 g fiber, 1,300 mg sodium, n/a g sugar

Choice That Sounds Good for You but Isn't

Chicken Marsala: 1,090 calories, 33 g protein, 76 g carbohydrates, 66 g total fat, 23 g saturated fat, n/a g trans fat, n/a mg cholesterol, 4 g fiber, 2,060 mg sodium, n/a g sugar

Your Favorite Mexican Restaurant

Best Meals

Chicken Fajitas: 851 calories, 56 g protein, 90 g carbohydrates, 29 g total fat, 6 g saturated fat, n/a g trans fat, 121 mg cholesterol, 6 g fiber, 2,002 mg sodium, 20 g sugar

Chicken Enchiladas (2): 501 calories, 41 g protein, 16 g carbohydrates, 24 g total fat, 10 g saturated fat, n/a g trans fat, 116 mg cholesterol, 3 g fiber, 1,469 mg sodium, 10 g sugar

Worst Choice

Taco Beef Nachos: 1,625 calories, 70 g protein, 85 g carbohydrates, 113 g total fat, 55 g saturated fat, n/a g trans fat, 242 mg cholesterol, 14 g fiber, 3,308 mg sodium, 22 g sugar

Choice That Sounds Good for You but Isn't

Traditional Beef Taco Salad: 1,291 calories, 57 g protein, 94 g carbohydrates, 80 g total fat, 29 g saturated fat, n/a g trans fat, 126 mg cholesterol, 19 g fiber, 2,033 mg sodium, 9 g sugar

Chapter 8

EAT THIS, NOT THAT

Make the Right Choice Every Time

WHEN IT COMES TO THE ABS DIET, I'm all about cheating. One meal a week, eat whatever you want. Not only has a cheat meal been shown to rev your metabolism (if you keep it in check), it also does something that's a little less tangible. It keeps your cravings at bay, reminds you that you're not denied all of your favorite foods, and gives you the strength to dig in and eat right for the rest of the week. (Many people say they don't even crave the cheat meal after a while.) That said, I also think you can make smart decisions when you're indulging. After all, if you make a good choice at your cheat meal, you may save yourself zillions of calories and fat, without sacrificing even a hint of taste. For that reason, I want you to be equipped with good information about dozens of nutritional dilemmas so you're able to make good decisions anytime and anyplace—in many cases, being able to choose the lesser of two evils. Remember, the journey to a great body is about making smart decisions at every intersection.

Bagel

Eat this: *Einstein Bros. Wild Blueberry Bagel with 2 Tbsp reduced-fat cream cheese* 410 calories, 12 g protein, 79 g carbohydrates, 6 g total fat, 3.5 g saturated fat, 3 g fiber, 595 mg sodium
Not that: *Panera Bread Blueberry Bagel with 2 oz reduced-fat cream*

cheese 470 calories, 17 g protein, 71 g carbohydrates, 14.5 g total fat, 8 g saturated fat, 4 g fiber, 770 mg sodium
Why: Panera bagel's higher protein and lower carb makeup would push it past the Einstein Bros. bagel—if it didn't have more than double the saturated fat.

Ballpark Foods

Eat this: *Hot dog with mustard and sauerkraut, 16 oz light beer, soft pretzel* 727 calories, 21 g fat, 18 g protein
Not that: *Chili dog, 16 oz regular beer, cheese nachos* 860 calories, 37 g fat, 24 g protein
Why: Go light, or the only thing stretching in the seventh inning will be your pants.

Banana Split

Eat this: *Dairy Queen Banana Split* 530 calories, 8 g protein, 98 g carbohydrates, 14 g total fat, 10 g saturated fat, 3 g fiber, 180 mg sodium
Not that: *Baskin-Robbins Banana Split Sundae* 1,030 calories, 12 g protein, 168 g carbohydrates, 39 g total fat, 23 g saturated fat, 7 g fiber, 190 mg sodium
Why: A DQ split is 34 percent smaller than one from Baskin-Robbins and has nearly half the calories and saturated fat.

Breakfast, Diner

Eat this: *8 oz lean top round steak, 2 scrambled eggs, 1 slice whole-wheat toast with jam* 791 calories, 30 g fat, 97 g protein, 26 g carbohydrates
Not that: *3 links sausage, 1 stack of three 6" pancakes with 1 pat butter and 2 Tbsp syrup* 901 calories, 48.5 g fat, 27 g protein, 91 g carbohydrates
Why: Pack in Powerfoods with lean meat and eggs over processed meat and white flour.

Breakfast Sandwich

Eat this: *Burger King Ham, Egg & Cheese Croissan'wich* 340 calories, 18 g protein, 26 g carbohydrates, 18 g total fat, 6 g saturated fat, 1 g fiber, 1,230 mg sodium
Not that: *Hardee's Ham, Egg, and Cheese Biscuit* 560 calories, 23 g

protein, 37 g carbohydrates, 35 g total fat, 10 g saturated fat, 0 g fiber, 1,800 mg sodium

Why: The BK version has more than 200 fewer calories and almost half the fat.

Burrito

Eat this: *Baja Fresh Steak Burrito* 850 calories, 49 g protein, 67 g carbohydrates, 46 g total fat, 18 g saturated fat, 7 g fiber, 2,260 mg sodium

Not that: *Chipotle Steak Fajita Burrito* 1,035 calories, 51 g protein, 110 g carbohydrates, 44 g total fat, 15 g saturated fat, 8 g fiber, 3,006 mg sodium

Why: Baja Fresh is clearly the lesser of two evils, considering Chipotle's higher carbs and sky-high sodium content.

Chicken, Fast-Food

Eat this: *Boston Market ¼ White Rotisserie Chicken (skinless) with Garlic Dill New Potatoes and Green Beans* 410 calories, 47 g protein, 37 g carbohydrates, 8.5 g total fat, 3 g saturated fat, 6 g fiber, 940 mg sodium

Not that: *KFC Two-Piece (breast and drumstick) Meal with Mashed Potatoes, Gravy, and Green Beans* 680 calories, 54 g protein, 37 g carbohydrates, 35 g total fat, 9 g saturated fat, 3 g fiber, 2,500 mg sodium

Why: With less than half the fat and sodium and twice the fiber, New England rotisserie sacks Southern fried.

Chicken, Fried

Eat this: *KFC Snacker Sandwich* 320 calories, 14 g protein, 29 g carbohydrates, 17 g total fat, 3 g saturated fat, 2 g fiber, 690 mg sodium

Not that: *Chick-fil-A Chicken Sandwich* 410 calories, 28 g protein, 38 g carbohydrates, 16 g total fat, 3.5 g saturated fat, 1 g fiber, 1,300 mg sodium

Why: The Colonel wins the battle of calories and sodium.

Chicken Salad

Eat this: *Così Bombay Chicken Salad with Peppercorn Ranch Dressing* 438 calories, 29 g protein, 15 g carbohydrates, 31 g total

fat, n/a g saturated fat, 4 g fiber, 896 mg sodium
Not that: *Panera Grilled Chicken Caesar Salad* 560 calories,
39 g protein, 26 g carbohydrates, 34 g total fat, 9 g saturated
fat, 4 g fiber, 1,270 mg sodium
Why: Cosí gets the nod, with less calories, carbs, fat, and
sodium than Panera's glorified Caesar.

Chicken Taco

Eat this: *Baja Fresh Charbroiled Chicken Baja Tacos (2)*
420 calories, 24 g protein, 56 g carbohydrates, 10 g total
fat, 2 g saturated fat, 4 g fiber, 460 mg sodium
Not that: *Taco Bell Ranchero Chicken Tacos, Fresco Style (2)*
340 calories, 24 g protein, 42 g carbohydrates, 8 g total fat,
3 g saturated fat, 6 g fiber, 1,460 mg sodium
Why: Despite having the same low-calorie, high-protein
balance as the Baja Fresh tacos, Taco Bell's are drenched
in sodium.

Chinese Takeout

Eat this: *Panda Express Kung Pao Chicken and Mixed
Veggies* 330 calories, 18 g protein, 20 g carbohydrates,
22 g total fat, 4 g saturated fat, 8 g fiber, 650 mg sodium
Not that: *Manchu Wok Kung Pao Chicken and Mixed
Vegetables* 372 calories, 8 g protein, 22 g carbohydrates,
28 g total fat, 4 g saturated fat, 4 g fiber, 730 mg sodium
Why: Panda wins the Kung Pao throwdown with twice
the protein and fiber and less fat than Manchu Wok.

Fish Sandwich

Eat this: *McDonald's Filet-O-Fish (with tartar sauce, no
cheese)* 350 calories, 14 g protein, 37 g carbohydrates,
16 g total fat, 4 g saturated fat, 2 g fiber, 550 mg sodium
Not that: *Burger King Big Fish Sandwich (with tartar sauce,
no cheese)* 630 calories, 24 g protein, 67 g carbohydrates,
30 g total fat, 6 g saturated fat, 4 g fiber, 1,380 mg sodium
Why: Throw the BK fish back—it has nearly twice the fat,
more than twice the sodium, and 280 more calories.

Fruit Drink

Eat this: *Dunkin' Donuts Strawberry Fruit Coolatta (16 oz)* 290 calories, 0 g protein, 72 g carbohydrates, 0 g total fat, 0 g saturated fat, 1 g fiber, 30 mg sodium

Not that: *Krispy Kreme Berries & Kreme Chiller (12 oz)* 620 calories, 3 g protein, 92 g carbohydrates, 28 g total fat, 24 g saturated fat, <1 g fiber, 220 mg sodium

Why: Half the calories and zero fat, the DD drink is the cool choice.

Halloween Candy

Eat this: *Hershey's Special Dark Nuggets with Almonds (1 piece)* 55 calories, 3.5 g total fat, 1.5 g saturated fat

Bit-O-Honey (6 pieces) 170 calories, 3 g total fat, 2 g saturated fat

Whoppers (9 pieces) 90 calories, 3.5 g total fat, 3.5 g saturated fat

Not that: *Caramels (4 pieces)* 154 calories, 3 g total fat, 1 g saturated fat

Candy Corn (12 pieces) 70 calories

Werther's Original Hard Candies (6 pieces) 120 calories, 26 g carbohydrates, 2 g total fat, 2 g saturated fat, 120 mg sodium

Why: Dark chocolate helps lower LDL (bad) cholesterol; our Powerfood friend, the almond (in the nuggets and Bit-O-Honey), also helps the heart and lowers cholesterol; and malted milk balls provide a low-cal chocolate fix. They all certainly trump pure sugar.

Happy Hour

Eat this: *Chicken fingers (4)* 640 calories, 31 g protein, 42 g carbohydrates, 38 g total fat, 8 g saturated fat

Not that: *Nachos with cheese and jalapeño peppers (9–12 chips)* 912 calories, 21 g protein, 90 g carbohydrates, 51 g total fat, 20 g saturated fat

Why: Though bathed in fat, at least there's some chicken in those fingers.

Ice Cream

Eat this: *Baskin-Robbins Banana Nut (4 oz scoop)* 260 calories, 5 g protein, 27 g carbohydrates, 16 g total fat, 7 g saturated fat, 1 g fiber, 75 mg sodium

Not that: *Cold Stone Creamery banana ice cream with nuts (6 oz scoop)* 370 calories, 6 g protein, 40 g carbohydrates, 22 g total fat, 14 g saturated fat, 0 g fiber, 85 mg sodium

Why: Even if you leave those 2 extra ounces in the cone (yeah, right), Cold Stone's rich ingredients tax your waistline.

Noodles

Eat this: *P.F. Chang's Singapore Street Noodles* 570 calories, 28 g protein, 91 g carbohydrates, 16 g total fat, 1.5 g saturated fat, 38 g fiber, 2,238 g sodium

Not that: *Chili's Grilled Shrimp Alfredo* 1,540 calories, 77 g protein, 123 g carbohydrates, 84 g total fat, 40 g saturated fat, 6 g fiber, 3,170 mg sodium

Why: With a third of the calories and a fifth of the fat, Chang's ode to Asia trounces Chili's cream- and butter-based Italian gut bomb.

Panini

Eat this: *Atlanta Bread Company Turkey Club Panini (with bacon)* 750 calories, 42 g protein, 83 g carbohydrates, 27 g total fat, 9 g saturated fat, 4 g fiber, 1,990 mg sodium

Not that: *Panera Smokehouse Turkey Panini (with bacon) on Artisan Three Cheese Bread* 840 calories, 51 g protein, 77 g carbohydrates, 37 g total fat, 15 g saturated fat, 5 g fiber, 2,770 mg sodium

Why: Even with bacon on both sandwiches, Panera's version weighs in with nearly two times the saturated fat and enough sodium to preserve a small city.

Pizza

Eat this: *Domino's medium cheese pizza on Classic Hand-Tossed crust (1 slice)* 210 calories, 9 g protein, 30 g carbohydrates, 8 g total fat, 3 g saturated fat, 1 g fiber, 335 mg sodium

Not that: *Pizza Hut medium cheese Hand-Tossed Style Pizza (1 slice)* 230 calories, 12 g protein, 25 g carbohydrates, 10 g total fat, 4.5 g saturated fat, 1 g fiber, 620 mg sodium

Why: Have more than a slice or two, and the calorie and fat difference becomes exponential.

Pizza, Personal

Eat this: *Taco Bell Mexican Pizza* 530 calories, 20 g protein, 46 g carbohydrates, 30 g total fat, 8 g saturated fat, 6 g fiber, 1,000 mg sodium

Not that: *Pizza Hut Personal Pan Supreme Pizza* 710 calories, 32 g protein, 70 g carbohydrates, 34 g total fat, 13 g saturated fat, 4 g fiber, 1,800 mg sodium

Why: Both mix meat, vegetables, and crisp crusts, but the Italian version is weighed down with almost 200 more calories, 5 g more saturated fat, and 800 mg more sodium.

Root Beer Float

Eat this: *A&W Root Beer Float (medium, 20 oz)* 330 calories, 2 g protein, 77 g carbohydrates, 5 g total fat, 3 g saturated fat, 0 g fiber, 105 mg sodium

Not that: *Sonic Float (large, 20 oz)* 440 calories, 5 g protein, 80 g carbohydrates, 12 g total fat, 7 g saturated fat, 0 g fiber, 160 mg sodium

Why: A&W has 110 fewer calories and less than half the fat.

Salad, Fast-Food

Eat this: *McDonald's Asian Salad with Grilled Chicken* 300 calories, 32 g protein, 23 g carbohydrates, 10 g total fat, 1 g saturated fat, 5 g fiber, 890 mg sodium

Not that: *Wendy's Mandarin Chicken Salad* 550 calories, 29 g protein, 53 g carbohydrates, 26 g total fat, 3 g saturated fat, 6 g fiber, 1,230 mg sodium

Why: Do you want extra fat, calories, and carbohydrates in a salad?

Steak

Eat this: *Outback Steakhouse 14 oz Rib-Eye* 730 calories, 92 g protein, 0 g carbohydrates, 40 g total fat, 0 g fiber, n/a mg sodium

Not that: *Chili's Flame-Grilled Ribeye* 960 calories, 40 g protein, 1 g carbohydrates, 87 g total fat, 0 g fiber, 1,090 mg sodium

Why: Outback's formidable rib eye wins with less than half the fat and more than twice the protein of Chili's steak.

Sushi

Eat this: *9 California rolls, 6 pieces salmon nigiri, 1 c miso soup* 804 calories, 10 g total fat, 28 g protein

Not that: *9 orange rolls, 1 spicy shrimp hand roll (cone-shaped roll), 1½ c salad with ginger-sesame dressing* 1,262 calories, 32 g total fat, 59.5 g protein

Why: Even fish can cost you a lot if it's dressed up too much.

Turkey Sandwich, Part I

Eat this: *Wendy's Roasted Turkey & Swiss Frescata* 480 calories, 25 g protein, 52 g carbohydrates, 20 g total fat, 6 g saturated fat, 4 g fiber, 1,520 mg sodium

Not that: *Arby's Market Fresh Roast Turkey Ranch & Bacon* 834 calories, 49 g protein, 73 g carbohydrates, 38 g total fat, 11 g saturated fat, 4 g fiber, 2,258 mg sodium

Why: Wendy's Frescata trounces Arby's Market Fresh catastrophe, with significantly less calories, fat, carbs, and sodium.

Turkey Sandwich, Part II

Eat this: *Subway 6-inch Turkey Breast sub on wheat with Swiss cheese, lettuce, tomatoes, onions, green peppers, olives and pickles, honey mustard, and mayo* 360 calories, 22 g protein, 53 g carbohydrates, 9 g total fat, 4 g saturated fat, 4 g fiber, 1,145 mg sodium

Not that: *Arby's Market Fresh Roast Turkey & Swiss Sandwich (includes green leaf lettuce, sliced tomatoes, red onion rings, mayo, and spicy brown honey mustard on honey wheat bread)* 725 calories, 44 g protein, 73 g carbohydrates, 30 g total fat, 8 g saturated fat, 4 g fiber, 1,788 mg sodium

Why: A brown bag from Arby's packs more than three times the fat, double the calories, and more sodium.

Wrap, Spicy

Eat this: *Chick-fil-A Spicy Chicken Cool Wrap* 410 calories, 35 g protein, 44 g carbohydrates, 12 g total fat, 3.5 g saturated fat, 8 g fiber, 1,340 mg sodium

Not that: *Taco Bell Spicy Chicken Crunchwrap Supreme* 540 calories, 19 g protein, 67 g carbohydrates, 23 g total fat, 7 g saturated fat, 4 g fiber, 1,360 mg sodium

Why: Chick-fil-A's spicy wrap delivers the heat with nearly twice the protein and half of the fat.

MORE SMOOTH MOVES!

New Smoothie Recipes for On-the-Go Eating

IF YOU'VE SPENT ANY TIME at all spinning through the Abs Diet series, then you know my take on the smoothie. It's the all-powerful master key that frees you from the things that handcuff you to your weight. Why? Because it smacks your dietary excuses upside the head. You say you love dessert too much to stick to a diet? Well, you can make good-for-you smoothies that are sweeter than a puppy's face. You're always hungry when you try dieting? A smoothie will fill your tank up so well that you're never going to be tempted to ruin your efforts with chips, dips, or Cool Whips. No time to make breakfast? Ha. Throw the ingredients in a blender, and you've got a Powerfood-packed meal that's the second best way to start any day.

You've likely seen the dozens of other smoothie recipes I've shared in the Abs Diet series, but you know what I say: Smoothies are like wine—there are infinite nuances of flavors, so why not appreciate them all? (Thought I was going to say "wine and women," didn't you?) In that spirit, here's to serving up some more ideas for blended perfection.

The Ultimate Smoothie Selector

WHEN YOU BECOME A SMOOTHIE AFICIONADO, you have to think of yourself like a bartender, with a shelf full of different ingredients that can be combined in thousands of ways to make different drinks. But instead of hard liquor, fruit juices, and cheese-stuffed olives, your bar is stocked with Powerfoods that'll keep you satisfied, help you build muscle, and deliver nutrients that will make you leaner and healthier at the same time. Below, here's what you should stock in your smoothie bar. Experiment with combinations on your own, or use one of the recipes that follow.

Peanut butter: Packed with protein, manganese, and niacin, peanuts can help stave off heart disease and promote weight loss.

Fat-free milk: You get all the calcium and protein, none of the fat.

Low-fat vanilla yogurt: Every scoop packs lots of calcium and digestion-aiding probiotics.

Fat-free chocolate frozen yogurt: Calcium, phosphorus, and none of the guilt.

Raspberries: Antioxidant powerhouses bursting with fiber, manganese, and vitamin C, these berries will keep your heart and brain in top shape.

Blueberries: Their huge amounts of antioxidants, such as anthocyanins, have been shown to slow brain decline and reverse memory loss.

Whey protein: Its essential amino acids help pack on muscle—and thus burn fat.

Cherries: In addition to providing vitamin C and fiber, cherries have been linked to reducing arthritis pain.

Bananas: Heavy on potassium, fiber, and vitamin B_6, bananas do wonders for your heart and provide good carbs to keep you full and energized.

Frozen mangoes: To their stock of vitamins A and C, mangoes add a healthy dose of beta-carotene, which helps prevent cancer and promotes healthy skin.

Pineapple-orange juice: OJ has vitamin C, and pineapple contains bromelain, a cancer-inhibiting, inflammation-reducing enzyme.

Ice: Adds bulk to smoothies—calorie-free.

Your creativity and tastebuds may dictate what ingredients you'll match (chocolate and cherry, perhaps?). Or for ideas, use one of these smoothies made from the base list of ingredients.

PROCESS MAKES PERFECT

The only at-home meal that's simpler than a smoothie is a piece of fruit. Still, that doesn't mean you can't appreciate the finer points of making these creamy concoctions. These tips will make sure your blender renders the perfect meal.

▶ **The blender:** You need one with a powerful motor (at least 400 watts) to handle chopping ice and shredding fruit.

▶ **The ingredients:** For best results, use a combination of frozen and fresh fruit. Frozen fruits lend thickness, while bananas add creaminess.

▶ **The order:** Pour in the liquid ingredients first for accurate measurements and a good consistency, then add the chunkier stuff.

▶ **The timing:** The less blending, the better. If you blend too long, it'll taste like paste. Treat your blender like any annoying co-worker: Don't let it go on for too long before you put an end to all the noise.

Throw Fruit for a Loop

1   cup pineapple
1   cup ice
½   cup fresh or frozen blueberries
½   cup fresh or frozen raspberries
½   cup low-fat vanilla yogurt

Combine all the ingredients in a blender and blend until smooth.

Serves 1

Nutritional information, per smoothie: 252 calories, 8 g protein, 54 g carbs, 2 g total fat, 1 g saturated fat, 8 g fiber, 85 mg sodium

Tea It Up

3   tablespoons water
1   green tea bag
2   teaspoons honey
1½   cups frozen blueberries
½   medium banana
¾   cup light vanilla soy milk

In small glass measuring cup or bowl, microwave the water on high until steaming hot. Add the tea bag and brew for 3 minutes. Remove the tea bag. Stir the honey into the tea until it dissolves. In a blender with ice-crushing ability, combine the berries, banana, and milk, then add the tea and blend everything together.

Serves 1

Nutritional information, per smoothie: 296 calories, 5 g protein, 68 g carbs, 3 g total fat, 0 g saturated fat, 8 g fiber, 76 mg sodium

Reese's into Pieces

1   cup fat-free milk
1   banana
½   cup fat-free chocolate frozen yogurt
⅓   cup whey protein
2   tablespoons peanut butter

Combine all the ingredients in a blender and blend until smooth.

Serves 1

Nutritional information, per smoothie: 694 calories, 76 g protein, 69 g carbs, 20 g total fat, 4 g saturated fat, 6 g fiber, 379 mg sodium

Tropical Paradise

1   cup pineapple-OJ
1   cup ice
½   cup pitted cherries
½   cup fresh or frozen mango chunks
½   cup low-fat vanilla yogurt

Combine all the ingredients in a blender and blend until smooth.

Serves 1

Nutritional information, per smoothie: 393 calories, 11 g protein, 89 g carbs, 2 g total fat, 1 g saturated fat, 3 g fiber, 92 mg sodium

Beachside Blend

1   cup pineapple-OJ
1   cup ice
½   cup fresh or frozen blueberries
½   cup fresh or frozen mango chunks

Combine all the ingredients in a blender and blend until smooth.

Serves 1

Nutritional information, per smoothie: 220 calories, 4 g protein, 54 g carbs, 0.5 g total fat, 0 g saturated fat, 3 g fiber, 11 mg sodium

Even More Ideas!

IN THEORY, you can take any combination of healthful ingredients, put them in a blender, and come up with your own Powerfood smoothie. (How do you think they came up with V8?) Now, it's not going to work all the time (green beans and oatmeal, probably not). But there are enough combinations of great ingredients to make sure you never get bored with trying new equations. In fact, several members of our Abs Diet online forums make it their mission to come up with great new combinations that they share with other Abs Diet devotees. Here are even more examples of great smoothie recipes.

Real Almond Joy

½   up plain nonfat yogurt
1   medium banana
1   tablespoon almond butter
¾   cup orange juice
Dash of cinnamon

In a blender, combine the yogurt, banana, almond butter, and orange juice. Blend until smooth. Sprinkle with cinnamon.

Serves 1

Nutritional information, per smoothie: 338 calories, 10 g protein, 59 g carbs, 10 g total fat, 1 g saturated fat, 4 g fiber, 141 mg sodium

Catch Some Flax

2   cups fresh or unsweetened frozen raspberries
6   ounces fat-free vanilla yogurt
4   tablespoons calcium-fortified orange juice
1   tablespoon flax meal or flaxseed
1   tablespoon wheat germ

Combine all the ingredients in a blender and blend until smooth.

Serves 1

Nutritional information, per smoothie: 271 calories, 8 g protein, 53 g carbs, 5.5 g total fat, 0 g saturated fat, 19 g fiber, 3 mg sodium

The Lean Luau

½   cup low-fat vanilla yogurt
½   cup drained pineapple chunks
½   teaspoon pure vanilla extract
¼   cup fat-free milk
8   ice cubes

Combine all the ingredients in a blender and blend until smooth.

Serves 1

Nutritional information, per smoothie: 185 calories, 9 g protein, 34 g carbs, 1.5 g total fat, 1 g saturated fat, 1 g fiber, 111 mg sodium

Are You Nuts?

½   cup light vanilla soy milk
½   cup frozen raspberries
½   cup frozen blueberries
½   banana
2   tablespoons chopped almonds
1   teaspoon pure vanilla extract

Combine all the ingredients in a blender and blend until smooth.

Serves 1

Nutritional information, per smoothie: 308 calories, 8 g protein, 55 g carbs, 8 g total fat, 0.5 g saturated fat, 10 g fiber, 49 mg sodium

Crandaddy of Them All

8   unsweetened frozen strawberries (about 1 cup)
1   medium banana
¼   cup unsweetened frozen cranberries
½   cup low-fat milk
2   teaspoons vanilla whey protein powder
1–2 teaspoons honey

In a blender, combine the strawberries, banana, cranberries, milk, and protein powder. Blend on high speed until smooth. Stir in the honey to taste.

Serves 1

Nutritional information, per smoothie: 271 calories, 12 g protein, 57 g carbs, 2 g total fat, 1 g saturated fat, 7 g fiber, 69 mg sodium

Liquid Sandwich

1   cup fat-free milk
1   banana
½   cup raspberries
½   cup fat-free frozen yogurt
1   tablespoon peanut butter

Combine all the ingredients in a blender and blend until smooth.

Serves 1

Nutritional information, per smoothie: 410 calories, 19 g protein, 69 g carbs, 9 g total fat, 2 g saturated fat, 8 g fiber, 242 mg sodium

NEW ABS DIET CIRCUITS

Workouts That Will Boost Your Metabolism and Burn Fat Fast

AS YOU READ IN CHAPTER 2, lots of things are responsible for boosting your metabolism—namely, those six powerful meals you're eating every day. Another great way to step on the metabolic accelerator is to make sure that you're doing the right kinds of exercise. Adding muscle will, in essence, give your fat a death sentence and banish it from your body forever. That's because it takes your body 50 times more calories to maintain that muscle than it does to maintain fat, so just by adding muscle, you're boosting your natural metabolic rate.

And that's only the beginning. I could go on and on about why exercise needs to be part of your Abs Diet repertoire. But for now, I'll pepper you with just a few compelling reasons.

▶ Exercise serves as a constant motivator to eat well and live healthy. In fact, research shows that guys who skip a workout due to "lack of time" are 76 percent less likely to maintain their weight loss.

▶ Exercise decreases stress (one of the main causes of overeating and diet ditching). In a Danish study, researchers found that those who exercise for 2 hours a week—about 17 minutes a day—are 61 percent less likely to feel highly stressed than sedentary people.

▶ Exercise puts your belly fat in the crosshairs. The research: Burning 1,100 calories a week through exercise prevents the accumulation of dangerous belly fat. In a Duke study, scientists tracked levels of visceral adipose tissue—the type of abdominal flab that causes high blood sugar, hypertension, and arterial inflammation. Those who burned 1,100 calories weekly didn't gain any of the deadly fat, while nonexercisers increased their belly-fat stores by 9 percent. Best of all, those 1,100 calories can be taken care of in just a few circuit workouts, which, whaddaya know, is exactly what the Abs Diet Workout entails. Add in a little more exercise, and you gain another huge benefit. People who burned an additional 550 calories per week reduced their visceral fat levels by 7 percent.

Before we get to the two new programs, here's a quick recap of what you should include in your weekly workout plan.

Strength training with circuits (three times a week): Resistance exercises add that muscle, which will burn fat. In Abs Diet circuits, you move from one exercise directly to another with little rest in between—keeping your heart rate up, burning more calories, and saving time. Focus on large muscle groups, especially your legs, so you add more calorie-frying muscle. More good news about strength exercises: University of Southern Maine researchers measured energy expenditure during exercise, and they found that weight training burns as many as 71 percent more calories than originally thought. In fact, they calculated that performing just one circuit of eight exercises can expend up to 231 calories. The more muscles you work, the more calories you'll burn.

High-intensity interval training (once a week): Instead of doing long, steady-state sessions of aerobic exercise, do one session per week of high-intensity intervals. The reason: Greater intensity not only boosts heart rate but has been shown to have a strong after-burn effect long after you finish your workout. After warming up, alternate periods of high-intensity and low-intensity cardiovascular work (such as 1 minute hard, then 1 minute slower, and so on). You can do it running, swimming, cycling, or using any cardiovascular machine.

Abdominal exercises (two or three times a week): Before a strength circuit, do a circuit of abs exercises (like crunches, the bicycle, and hanging knee raises) to strengthen your entire core. You'll build a strong foundation in your abdominals that you can show off—once you burn the fat.

You'll see countless ideas for circuits and programs in other books in the Abs Diet series, but here, as a bonus, are a few more—one tailored to someone who's just starting out, the other focusing on the advanced exerciser or athlete who can do more specialized moves.

New Workout
Abs Diet Circuit: Beginner

Perform each exercise for the amount of repetitions listed below, then move immediately to the next exercise with no more than 30 seconds of rest in between. Once you complete all the exercises, repeat. Start with two cycles and build up to three. Use light weight at first, adding more as you get stronger.

EXERCISE	REPETITIONS
Bench Press	10–12
Squat	12–15
Dumbbell Pullover	12–15
Overhead Lunge Walk	10–12 each leg
Dumbbell Cross Punch	12–15 each arm
Single-Leg Squat	8–12 each leg

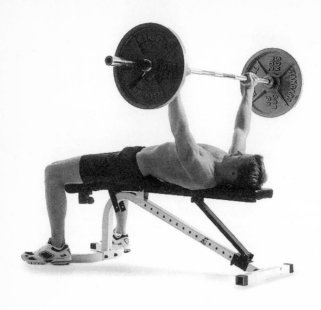

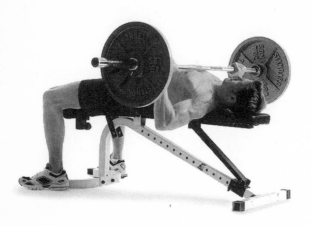

BENCH PRESS

Lie on your back on a flat bench with your feet on the floor. Grab the barbell with an overhand grip, your hands just beyond shoulder-width apart. Lift the bar off the uprights and hold it at arm's length over your chest. Slowly lower the bar to your chest. Pause, then push the bar back to the starting position.

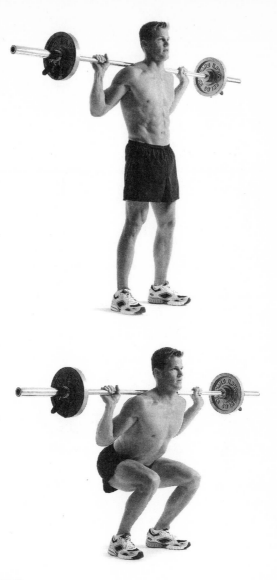

SQUAT

Hold a barbell with an overhand grip so that it rests comfortably on your upper back (or hold a dumbbell in each hand with your arms at your sides and your palms facing your outer thighs). Set your feet shoulder-width apart and keep your knees slightly bent, back straight, and eyes focused straight ahead. Slowly lower your body as if you were sitting back into a chair, keeping your back in its natural alignment and your lower legs nearly perpendicular to the floor. When your thighs are parallel to the floor, pause, then return to the starting position.

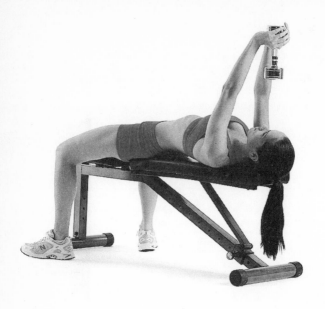

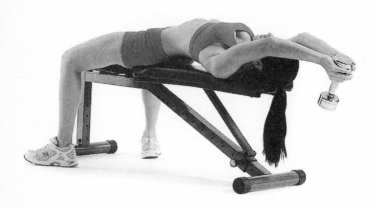

DUMBBELL PULLOVER

Grab a light dumbbell and lie flat on a bench. Wrapping your thumbs and forefingers in a diamond shape around the handle, use both hands to hold the weight vertically over your head. Keeping your elbows slightly bent, slowly lower the weight backward in an arc over your head until you feel a slight stretch in your sides and your upper arms are in line with your head. Pause, then slowly pull the weight back over your chest.

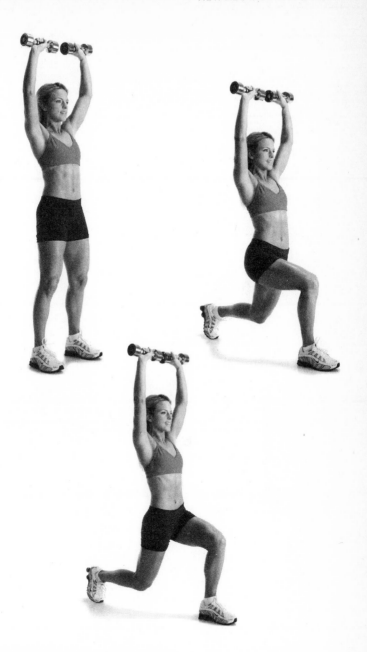

OVERHEAD LUNGE WALK

Hold a light barbell or two dumbbells at arm's length over your head, palms facing forward. Pull your abs in toward your spine to stabilize your core. Step one leg forward into a lunge, then press up and step forward into a lunge with your other leg. Keep walking for 10 to 12 lunges with each leg.

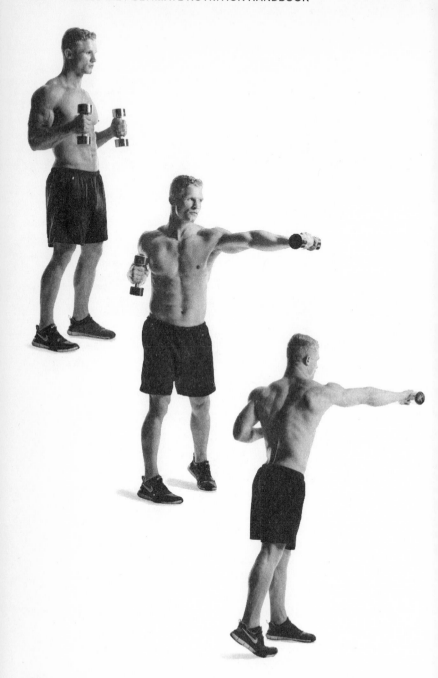

DUMBBELL CROSS PUNCH

Stand holding a pair of light dumbbells, palms angled in. Punch your
left fist forward and slightly to the right, rotating your wrist as you
go. Draw your arm back as you punch with your right fist.

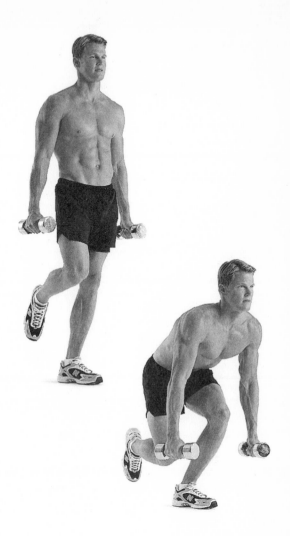

SINGLE-LEG SQUAT

Holding a dumbbell in each hand with your arms at your sides and your palms facing your outer thighs, stand with your knees slightly bent and your feet shoulder-width apart. Lift your right leg so that your knee is bent 90 degrees and your lower leg is parallel to the floor behind you. Slowly lower your body until your left thigh is parallel to the floor. Pause, then push your body back up to the starting position. Finish all of your repetitions on that side, then switch legs and repeat.

New Workout
Abs Diet Circuit: Athlete

Perform each exercise for the amount of repetitions listed below, then move immediately to the next exercise with no more than 30 seconds of rest in between. Once you complete all of the exercises, repeat. Start with two cycles and build up to three. Use light weight at first, adding more as you get stronger.

EXERCISE	REPETITIONS
Dumbbell Sumo Squat	12–15
Chinup	Maximum
Power Lateral Jump	12–15
Swiss Ball Pushup	12–15
Overhead Reverse Lunge	12–15
Cable Single-Arm Curl	10–12 each arm
Cable Incline-Bench Triceps Extension	10–12

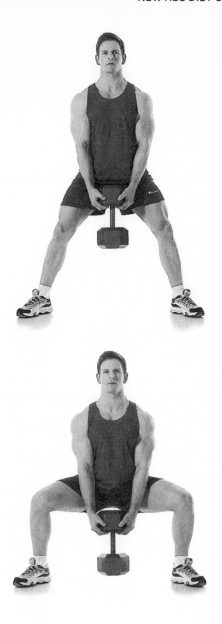

DUMBBELL SUMO SQUAT

Grab a heavy dumbbell and stand with your toes pointed out at 10 and 2 o'clock. Hold the weight with both hands at one end so the dumbbell points to the floor. Keeping your arms straight, lower your body until the end of the dumbbell nears the floor. Squeeze your glutes and push yourself back up to a standing position.

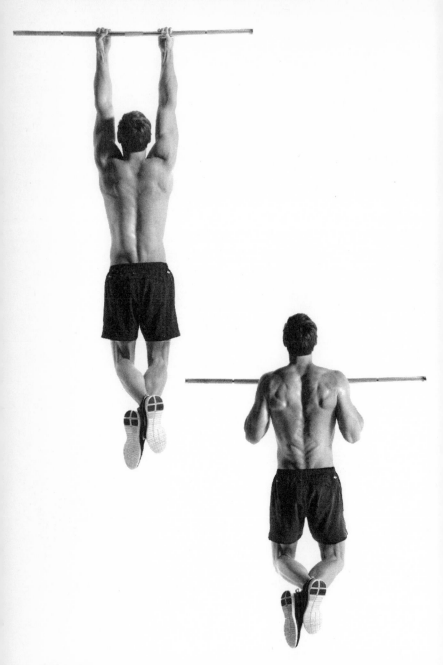

CHINUP

Grab a chinup bar with an underhand grip (palms toward you), your hands about shoulder-width apart. Pull yourself up until the bar is below your chin. Squeeze your biceps at the top, then slowly lower yourself until your arms are almost straight.

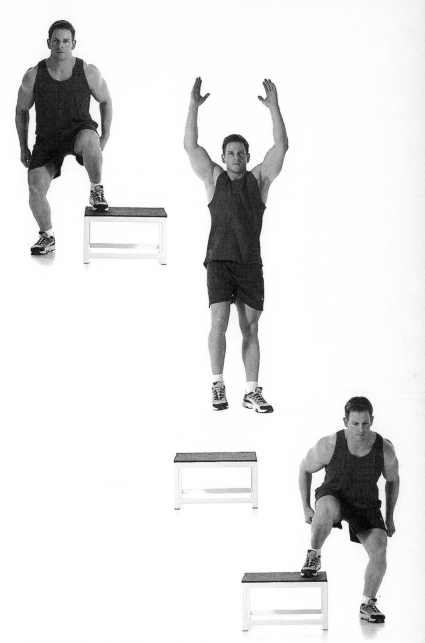

POWER LATERAL JUMP

Stand with your left foot on a step and your right foot on the floor. Dip slightly at the knees, then push off with enough force (swing your arms to help) to leave the floor. Land with your right foot on the step and your left foot on the floor. Repeat to the other side. That's one repetition.

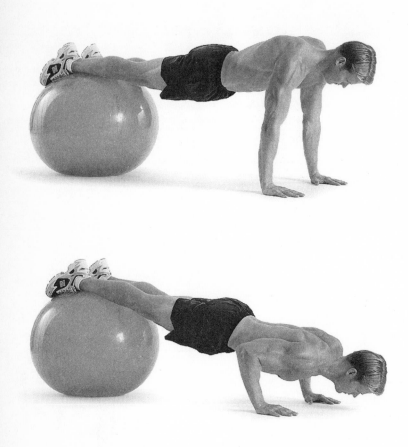

SWISS BALL PUSHUP

Get into a pushup position with your shins on a Swiss ball and your hands on the floor. Perform a traditional pushup by lowering your upper body toward the floor.

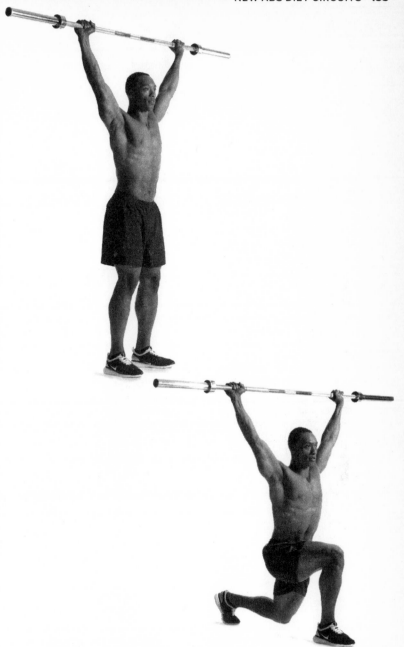

OVERHEAD REVERSE LUNGE

Grab a light barbell or broomstick with an overhand grip that's twice shoulder width. Holding the bar overhead with straight arms, step back with your left leg and lower your body until your right knee is bent 90 degrees. Push back to the starting position and repeat, this time stepping back with your right leg. That's one repetition.

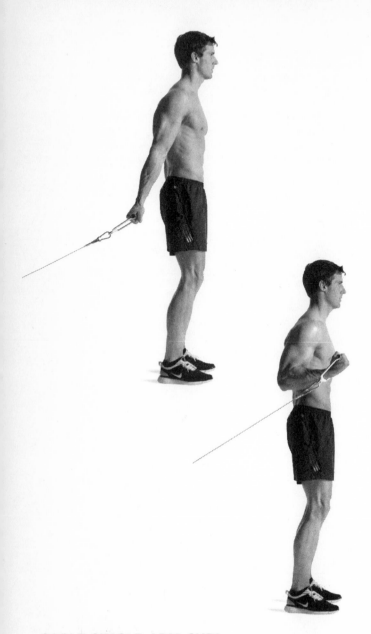

CABLE SINGLE-ARM CURL

Stand with your back to the weight stack of a cable station and grab the low-pulley handle with your right hand. Step forward so your right hand is a few inches behind you and your arm is straight. Keeping your elbow in place, curl the handle up until it reaches the side of your chest. Pause, then slowly return. Finish all of your repetitions on that side, then switch sides.

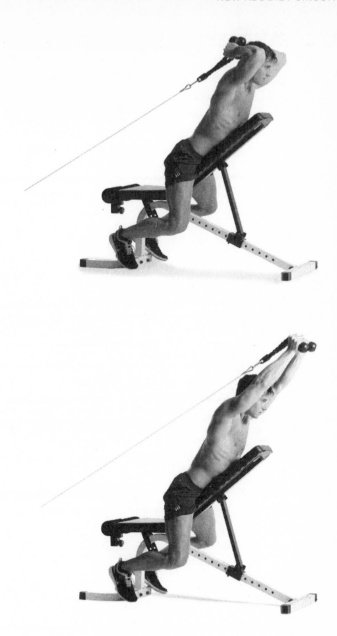

CABLE INCLINE-BENCH TRICEPS EXTENSION

Attach a rope to a low-pulley cable and place an incline bench a couple of feet in front of the pulley. Grab the rope and lie facedown on the bench with your arms straight and beside your ears. Without moving your upper arms, bend your elbows 90 degrees. Pause, then straighten your arms.

Bonus Abs Move!

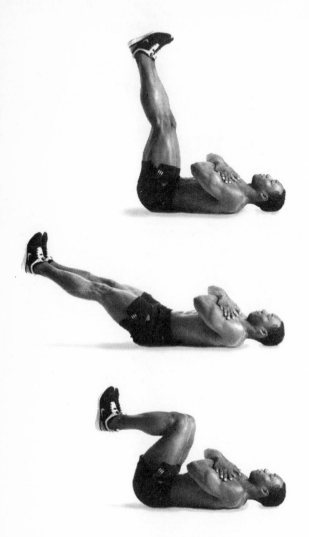

FLAT-BACK LEG-LOWERING DRILL

Lie on your back and raise your legs over your hips, with your knees slightly bent. Press the small of your back into the floor to eliminate the arch in your lower back. Keep your back in this position as you take 3 to 5 seconds to lower your legs. Upon reaching the lowest point at which you can still keep your back flat, bring your legs to your chest. Return to the starting position. Try to lower your legs more with each repetition. Do as many as you can.

Bonus Abs Move!

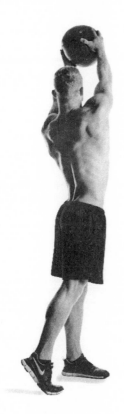

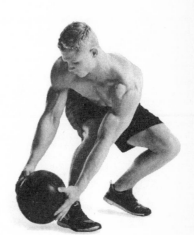

MEDICINE-BALL CHOP

Stand holding a medicine ball with your arms straight and over your left shoulder. Pivot to the left so that your right heel rises off the floor and your torso faces the left. This is the starting position. Quickly bend your knees and rotate your torso to the right as you draw your arms across your body and down. Once the ball is outside your right lower leg, quickly reverse the motion to return to the starting position, then switch positions to work the opposite side. Do 10 to 15 in each direction.

Appendix A

YOUR 14-DAY ABS DIET FOOD-AND-EXERCISE JOURNAL

With Motivational Secrets to Keep You Going

BY NOW, YOU KNOW THE RULES for losing weight: Eat the right foods, build some muscle, and let your body do the rest. No matter how well you know the formula, though, there are always more tricks, tips, and strategies to help you in your quest to lose your marshmallow middle. One of those tricks: Write down what you eat. It's not that anybody's going to check it, but being accountable to a piece of paper plays a huge deterrent role.

Here's the best part. You don't have to treat a food journal with the level of detail the IRS shows a 1099. A study at the University of Pittsburgh found that people who keep a basic food journal lose as much weight as those who record every single bite. It's following the process, not spelling out the details, that proves to be an effective way of staying under control. So instead of writing down weights or exact amounts, simply note what you ate and put a size next to it (S, M, or L should do). Once you get in the habit of doing it for a couple of weeks, you'll be well on your way to making your six Powerfood meals a habit. Use the space below (or any online food-recording program, if you prefer) to track your eating and exercise.

Day 1

Breakfast
_____

_____

Snack 1
_____

_____

Lunch
_____

_____

Snack 2
_____

_____

Dinner
_____

_____

Snack 3
_____

_____

Exercise
_____

_____

SIX-PACK SECRET

It's tempting to try to cram in more activities during the day, but don't sacrifice your pillow time to do so. People who sleep less weigh more. A Columbia University study showed that those who got only 6 hours of sleep a night were 23 percent more likely to be overweight than those who slept 7 to 9 hours.

Day 2

Breakfast
_____

_____

Snack 1
_____

_____

Lunch
_____

_____

Snack 2
_____

_____

Dinner
_____

_____

Snack 3
_____

_____

Exercise
_____

_____

SIX-PACK SECRET

Next time you're accused of twiddling your thumbs while your loved one is talking to you, say you're doing it for your health. A study by the Mayo Clinic found that fidgeting burns more calories than previously thought. When researchers equipped people with monitors that calculated slight levels of movement,

Day 3

Breakfast
_____

_____

Snack 1
_____

_____

Lunch
_____

_____

Snack 2
_____

_____

Dinner
_____

_____

Snack 3
_____

_____

Exercise
_____

_____

they found that overweight people simply moved less than lean people—and burned 350 fewer calories a day. The take-home: Any movement you can incorporate into your life—walking to the next office, tapping your foot while you're on the phone, juggling while having sex—will add to your weight-loss effort.

Day 4

Breakfast
_____

_____

Snack 1
_____

_____

Lunch
_____

_____

Snack 2
_____

_____

Dinner
_____

_____

Snack 3
_____

_____

Exercise
_____

_____

SIX-PACK SECRET

Maybe you see the doc only when you've got a case of strep throat or pinkeye (or pink anything, for that matter), but it wouldn't hurt you to schedule that physical you've been putting off. Researchers at Brown Medical School in Providence, Rhode Island, studied 900 formerly overweight people and concluded

Day 5

Breakfast
_____

_____

Snack 1
_____

_____

Lunch
_____

_____

Snack 2
_____

_____

Dinner
_____

_____

Snack 3
_____

_____

Exercise
_____

_____

that those whose weight loss was prompted by a medical con-
cern, such as a doctor's recommendation to lose weight,
dropped more pounds and proved better at keeping them off
than those who slimmed down for vanity reasons.

Day 6

Breakfast
_____

_____

Snack 1
_____

_____

Lunch
_____

_____

Snack 2
_____

_____

Dinner
_____

_____

Snack 3
_____

_____

Exercise
_____

_____

SIX-PACK SECRET

If you're a desk jockey, try to increase the amount of time
you spend out of the saddle. An Australian study found that
workers whose jobs require more than 6 hours of chair time a
day are up to 68 percent more likely to wind up overweight

Day 7

Breakfast
_____

_____

Snack 1
_____

_____

Lunch
_____

_____

Snack 2
_____

_____

Dinner
_____

_____

Snack 3
_____

_____

Exercise
_____

_____

or obese than those who sit less. Track your daily sit time for 3 days, then make an effort to cut 20 minutes off that number by going for a walk at lunch or heading down the hall instead of e-mailing colleagues.

Day 8

Breakfast

_____

Snack 1

_____

Lunch

_____

Snack 2

_____

Dinner

_____

Snack 3

_____

Exercise

_____

SIX-PACK SECRET

In the "who'd a thunk it?" category: Your khakis could play a role in weight loss. Wearing comfortable clothing to work may boost your daily calorie burn by 8 percent, according to a study at the University of Wisconsin–La Crosse. Using pedometers, researchers assessed whether the workday activity levels of

Day 9

Breakfast

_____

Snack 1

_____

Lunch

_____

Snack 2

_____

Dinner

_____

Snack 3

_____

Exercise

_____

people in a variety of professions bore any relationship to the clothing they wore. The finding: People took an average of 491 more steps on days they were more casually attired. It's more conducive to movement and less restrictive.

Day 10

Breakfast
_____

_____

Snack 1
_____

_____

Lunch
_____

_____

Snack 2
_____

_____

Dinner
_____

_____

Snack 3
_____

_____

Exercise
_____

_____

SIX-PACK SECRET

One of the biggest dietary pitfalls happens when you've got one hand on the remote and the other hand searching for something to occupy itself. Beware of boredom hunger—it's dictated by zoning out on the couch, not by what your stomach

Day 11

Breakfast _____

_____

Snack 1 _____

_____

Lunch _____

_____

Snack 2 _____

_____

Dinner _____

_____

Snack 3 _____

_____

Exercise _____

_____

is actually feeling. If you're reaching for something to eat out of habit, get up and take a walk—or brush your teeth and use mouthwash to kill your needless urge to feast.

Day 12

Breakfast
_____

_____

Snack 1
_____

_____

Lunch
_____

_____

Snack 2
_____

_____

Dinner
_____

_____

Snack 3
_____

_____

Exercise
_____

_____

SIX-PACK SECRET

We all know that the eyes are partly responsible for what goes into the stomach, but you can also use your eyes to keep stuff out. A University of Illinois at Urbana-Champaign study showed that people who spooned soup from bowls with unseen refilling devices ate 73 percent more than those whose bowls emptied as

Day 13

Breakfast
_____

_____

Snack 1
_____

_____

Lunch
_____

_____

Snack 2
_____

_____

Dinner
_____

_____

Snack 3
_____

_____

Exercise
_____

_____

they ate. The researchers say that doing something that reminds you of how much you've consumed—like keeping wrappers or bottle caps on your desk as visible evidence—will act as a deterrent for eating more.

Day 14

Breakfast

_____

Snack 1

_____

Lunch

_____

Snack 2

_____

Dinner

_____

Snack 3

_____

Exercise

_____

SIX-PACK SECRET

After studying 3,500 people from the National Weight Control Registry who maintained 60 or more pounds of weight loss for at least a year, researchers found that 44 percent weighed themselves every day. Don't rely solely on the scale to measure your progress, but it can be an early warning system.

Appendix B

FOOD BY THE NUMBERS

Comprehensive Nutritional Information for Your Food

THE ABS DIET IS ALL ABOUT centering your meals around the 12 Power-foods without worrying so much about numbers of calories, numbers of this, and numbers of that. It's most important to diversify your diet with protein, whole grains, healthy fats, and fruits and vegetables. That said, I know that accountants and fantasy football players aren't the only ones who like to look at numbers. That's why I'm including this chart of nutritional information: so those of you who do count calories or fat, for example, can see specifically how foods stack up. This information, from the USDA National Nutrient Database for Standard Reference—Release 18, isn't meant to make you worry about every single calorie you eat, but it does further your ultimate goal: having as much nutritional information as you need to make smart decisions every day.

BEANS AND LEGUMES

FOOD ITEM	SERVING SIZE	CALORIES
Baked beans	⅓ c	126
Baked beans, vegetarian	⅓ c	79
Bean sprouts (mung beans)	½ c	13
Black beans, cooked with salt	½ c	114
Black beans, dry	¼ c	165
Black-eyed peas, fresh	¼ c	33
Butter beans (lima), canned	½ c	95
Butter beans (lima), cooked with salt	½ c	105
Butter beans (lima), cooked without salt	½ c	105
Butter beans (lima), raw	½ c	88
Cannellini beans, cooked without salt	½ c	100
Cannellini beans, dry	¼ c	153
Chickpeas (garbanzo beans), cooked with salt	½ c	134
Chickpeas (garbanzo beans), cooked without salt	½ c	134
Edamame, frozen, prepared	½ c	95
Edamame (immature green soybeans), out of shell, cooked without salt	½ c	100
Falafel, cooked	2.25 in. patty	57
Falafel, dry	¼ c	120
French beans, cooked with salt	½ c	114
French beans, cooked without salt	½ c	114

PROTEIN (G)	CARB (G)	FIBER (G)	SUGAR (G)	FAT (G)	SAT FAT (G)	SODIUM (MG)
5	18	5	0	4	2	352
4	18	3	7	1	0	288
1	3	1	2	0	0	6
8	20	8	0	1	0	204
10	30	7	1	0	0	2
1	7	2	1	0	0	1
6	18	6	1	0	0	405
6	20	5	1	0	0	215
6	20	5	1	0	0	14
5	16	4	1	1	0	6
6	17	5	1	1	0	40
11	28	11	1	0	0	11
7	22	6	4	2	0	199
7	22	6	4	2	0	6
8	8	4	2	4	0	5
10	9	1	2	2.5	0	70
2	5	0	0	3	0	50
7	21	6	3	2	0	370
6	21	8	0	1	0	214
6	21	8	0	1	0	5

BEANS AND LEGUMES

FOOD ITEM	SERVING SIZE	CALORIES
French beans, raw	3 oz	30
Hummus	⅛ c	54
Kidney beans, red, cooked with salt	½ c	112
Kidney beans, red, cooked without salt	½ c	112
Lentils, brown, cooked with salt	½ c	115
Lentils, brown, cooked without salt	½ c	115
Navy beans, cooked with salt	½ c	127
Navy beans, cooked without salt	½ c	127
Pinto beans, cooked with salt	½ c	122
Pinto beans, cooked without salt	½ c	122
Refried beans, canned	½ c	118
Refried beans, fat-free	½ c	130
Refried beans, vegetarian	½ c	100
Soybeans, cooked	½ c	148
Soybeans, dry-roasted, salted	¼ c	194
Soybeans, dry-roasted, unsalted	¼ c	194
Soybeans, green, boiled without salt	½ c	127
White beans, small, cooked with salt	½ c	127

PROTEIN (G)	CARB (G)	FIBER (G)	SUGAR (G)	FAT (G)	SAT FAT (G)	SODIUM (MG)
2	6	2	0	0	0	0
1	6	1	0	3	0	74
8	20	7	0	0	0	211
8	20	7	0	0	0	2
9	20	8	2	0	0	236
9	20	8	2	0	0	2
7	24	10	0	1	0	216
7	24	10	0	1	0	0
8	22	8	0	1	0	203
8	22	8	0	1	0	1
7	20	7	0	2	1	379
6	18	6	1	0	0	580
6	17	6	2	1	0	560
14	8	5	3	7	1	1
17	14	4	0	9	1	70
17	14	4	0	9	1	1
11	10	4	0	6	1	13
8	23	9	0	1	0	213

BEVERAGES

FOOD ITEM	SERVING SIZE	CALORIES
Alcohol		
Beer, ale	12 fl oz	147
Beer, amber	12 fl oz	169
Beer, black and tan	12 fl oz	174
Beer, dark	12 fl oz	144
Beer, lager	12 fl oz	172
Beer, light	12 fl oz	103
Beer, nonalcoholic, O'Doul's	12 fl oz	70
Beer, pale ale	12 fl oz	179
Beer, porter	12 fl oz	190
Bloody Mary	8 fl oz	50
Bourbon, 80 proof	1.5 fl oz	98
Brandy, 80 proof	1.5 fl oz	96
Coffee and cream liqueur	1.5 fl oz	153
Coffee liqueur, 53 proof	1.5 fl oz	175
Coffee liqueur, 63 proof	1.5 fl oz	160
Crème de menthe	1.5 fl oz	186
Gin, 80 proof	1.5 fl oz	97
Gin, 100 proof	1.5 fl oz	124
Gin and tonic cocktail	6 fl oz	117
Highball cocktail	6 fl oz	111
Long Island iced tea	6 fl oz	142
Mai tai	1.5 fl oz	103
Manhattan cocktail	6 fl oz	213
Margarita	1.5 fl oz	94
Martini	1.5 fl oz	103
Piña colada	1.5 fl oz	82

PROTEIN (G)	CARB (G)	FIBER (G)	SUGAR (G)	FAT (G)	SAT FAT (G)	SODIUM (MG)
1	13	n/a	n/a	0	0	34
2	14	n/a	n/a	0	0	44
2	18	n/a	n/a	0	0	9
1	13	n/a	n/a	0	0	33
2	17	1	0	0	0	9
1	6	0	0	0	0	14
1	15	n/a	n/a	0	0	9
2	17	n/a	n/a	0	0	9
3	20	n	n/a	0	0	9
1	8	1	5	0	0	605
0	0	0	0	0	0	0
0	0	0	0	0	0	0
1	10	0	9	7	5	43
0	24	0	24	0	0	4
0	17	0	17	0	0	4
0	21	0	21	0	0	2
0	0	0	0	0	0	0
0	0	0	0	0	0	0
0	6	0	6	0	0	5
0	0	0	0	0	0	27
0	11	0	n/a	0	0	7
0	10	0	9	0	0	4
0	6	0	6	0	0	5
0	6	0	6	0	0	2
0	1	0	0	0	0	1
0	11	0	11	1	1	3

BEVERAGES

FOOD ITEM	SERVING SIZE	CALORIES
Rum, 80 proof	1.5 fl oz	97
Rum, 100 proof	1.5 fl oz	124
Sangria	5 fl oz	98
Screwdriver	6 fl oz	145
Tequila, 80 proof	1.5 fl oz	96
Tequila sunrise, canned	6 fl oz	205
Tom Collins cocktail	6 fl oz	69
Vodka, 80 proof	1.5 fl oz	97
Vodka, 100 proof	1.5 fl oz	124
Whiskey, 80 proof	1.5 fl oz	97
Whiskey sour cocktail, prepared with water, whiskey, and powder	6 fl oz	289
White Russian	1.5 fl oz	109
Wine cooler	5 fl oz	71
Wine, dessert, dry	5 fl oz	224
Wine, dessert, sweet	5 fl oz	236
Wine, dry, burgundy	5 fl oz	128
Wine, dry, claret	5 fl oz	127
Wine, dry, sherry	5 fl oz	102
Wine, light	5 fl oz	74
Wine, port	5 fl oz	236
Wine, red	5 fl oz	125
Wine, red, Merlot	5 fl oz	123
Wine, red, Pinot Noir	5 fl oz	122
Wine, red, Syrah	5 fl oz	123
Wine, red, Zinfandel	5 fl oz	131
Wine, white, Chenin Blanc	5 fl oz	120

PROTEIN (G)	CARB (G)	FIBER (G)	SUGAR (G)	FAT (G)	SAT FAT (G)	SODIUM (MG)
0	0	0	0	0	0	0
0	0	0	0	0	0	0
0	13	0	n/a	0	0	10
1	15	0	15	0	0	2
0	0	0	0	0	0	0
1	21	0	14	0	0	106
0	5	0	4	0	0	27
0	0	0	0	0	0	0
0	0	0	0	0	0	0
0	0	0	0	0	0	0
0	28	0	28	0	0	81
0	7	0	6	1	0	3
0	8	0	n/a	0	0	12
0	17	0	2	0	0	13
0	20	0	11	0	0	13
0	5	n/a	n/a	0	0	12
0	4	n/a	n/a	0	0	12
0	2	n/a	n/a	0	0	12
0	2	0	2	0	0	10
0	20	0	11	0	0	13
0	4	0	1	0	0	6
0	4	0	1	0	0	6
0	3	n	n/a	0	0	n/a
0	4	n/a	n/a	0	0	n/a
0	4	n/a	n/a	0	0	n/a
0	5	n/a	n/a	0	0	n/a

BEVERAGES

FOOD ITEM	SERVING SIZE	CALORIES
Wine, white, late harvest	5 fl oz	174
Wine, white, medium	5 fl oz	122
Wine, white, Pinot Grigio	5 fl oz	123
Wine, white, Sauvignon Blanc	5 fl oz	121
Wine spritzer	5 fl oz	59
Coffee and Tea		
Cappuccino, with 1% milk	8 fl oz	73
Chai, Celestial Seasonings, original	8 fl oz	0
Coffee, brewed	8 fl oz	2
Coffee, decaf, brewed	8 fl oz	0
Coffee, iced latte, with 1% milk	8 fl oz	60
Coffee, instant	1 Tbsp	5
Coffee, instant, decaf	1 Tbsp	12
Coffee, instant, 50% less caffeine	1 Tbsp	9
Coffee, latte, with 1% milk	8 fl oz	60
Coffee, mocha, with 1% milk	8 fl oz	200
Espresso	4 fl oz	11
Tea, black, decaf	8 fl oz	0
Tea, black, iced, unsweetened	8 fl oz	0
Juice		
Apple juice, unsweetened, bottled or canned	4 fl oz	58
Apple juice, unsweetened, frozen, prepared	4 fl oz	56
Apple-cranberry juice	4 fl oz	77
Cranberry juice, unsweetened	4 fl oz	58

PROTEIN (G)	CARB (G)	FIBER (G)	SUGAR (G)	FAT (G)	SAT FAT (G)	SODIUM (MG)
0	21	n/a	n/a	0	0	n/a
0	4	0	1	0	0	7
0	3	n/a	n/a	0	0	n/a
0	3	n	n/a	0	0	n/a
0	1	0	n/a	0	0	19
5	7	0	7	2	2	73
0	0	0	0	0	0	0
0	0	0	0	0	0	5
0	0	0	0	0	0	5
5	7	0	6	2	1	67
0	1	0	0	0	0	1
1	2	0	0	0	0	1
0	2	0	0	0	0	1
5	7	0	6	2	1	67
8	22	1	19	10	6	107
0	2	0	2	0	0	17
0	0	0	0	0	0	0
0	0	0	0	0	0	0
0	14	0	14	0	0	4
0	14	0	13	0	0	8
0	19	0	18	0	0	2
0	15	0	15	0	0	3

BEVERAGES

FOOD ITEM	SERVING SIZE	CALORIES
Cranberry juice cocktail	4 fl oz	68
Cranberry juice cocktail, low-calorie	4 fl oz	22
Grape juice, unsweetened	4 fl oz	77
Grape juice drink	4 fl oz	71
Grapefruit juice, unsweetened, canned, white	4 fl oz	47
Grapefruit juice white, unsweetened, frozen, from concentrate, prepared	4 fl oz	50
Grapefruit juice, white, raw	4 fl oz	48
Lemon juice, raw	4 fl oz	30
Lime juice, raw	4 fl oz	31
Orange juice, raw	4 fl oz	56
Orange juice, frozen, from concentrate, unsweetened, prepared	4 fl oz	56
Tomato juice, canned	4 fl oz	20
Tomato juice, canned, unsalted	4 fl oz	21
Tomato-vegetable juice, low-sodium	4 fl oz	27
Vegetable juice, V8	4 fl oz	25
Vegetable juice, V8, Picante	4 fl oz	25
Vegetable juice, V8, Spicy Hot	4 fl oz	25
Milk and Nondairy		
Half-and-half, fat-free	1 fl oz	18
Milk, fat-free, with added nonmilk fat solids	1 c	91
Milk, low fat 1%	1 c	118
Milk, reduced fat 2%	1 c	122

PROTEIN (G)	CARB (G)	FIBER (G)	SUGAR (G)	FAT (G)	SAT FAT (G)	SODIUM (MG)
0	17	0	15	0	0	3
0	5	0	5	0	0	4
1	19	0	19	0	0	4
0	18	0	18	0	0	11
1	11	0	11	0	0	1
1	12	0	12	0	0	1
1	11	0	11	0	0	1
0	10	0	3	0	0	1
1	10	0	2	0	0	2
1	13	0	10	0	0	1
1	13	0	10	0	0	1
1	5	1	4	0	0	323
1	5	0	4	0	0	12
1	6	1	5	0	0	85
1	5	1	4	0	0	240
1	5	1	4	0	0	295
1	5	1	4	0	0	355
1	3	0	1.5	0.5	0	43
9	12	0	12	0	0	130
10	14	0	11	3	2	143
8	11	0	12	5	3	100

BEVERAGES

FOOD ITEM	SERVING SIZE	CALORIES
Milk, whole	1 c	146
Soy milk	1 c	127

BREADS AND CRACKERS

FOOD ITEM	SERVING SIZE	CALORIES
Bagel, cinnamon-raisin	1 oz	77
Bagel, egg	1 oz	79
Bagel, onion	1 oz	78
Bagel, plain	1 oz	78
Bagel, poppy seed	1 oz	78
Bagel, whole-grain	1 oz	57
Biscuit, buttermilk, or plain prep. from recipe	½ of 2.5 in. biscuit	106
Biscuit, plain, or buttermilk commercially baked	½ of 2.5 in. biscuit	64
Bread, banana	½ slice (1 oz)	98
Bread, Ezekiel 4:9 Sprouted Grain Bread	1 slice (34 g)	80
Bread, French	1 slice (1 oz)	82
Bread, pita, white	½ of 6.5 in. pita (1 oz)	82
Bread, pita, whole-wheat	½ of 6.5 in. pita (1 oz)	85
Bread, pumpernickel	1 slice (1 oz)	71
Bread, raisin	1 slice (approx. 1 oz)	71
Bread, rye	1 slice (approx. 1 oz)	83
Bread, seven-grain	1 slice (approx. 1 oz)	65

PROTEIN (G)	CARB (G)	FIBER (G)	SUGAR (G)	FAT (G)	SAT FAT (G)	SODIUM (MG)
8	11	0	13	8	5	98
11	12	3	1	5	1	135

PROTEIN (G)	CARB (G)	FIBER (G)	SUGAR (G)	FAT (G)	SAT FAT (G)	SODIUM (MG)
3	16	1	2	0	0	91
3	15	1	n/a	1	0	143
3	15	1	n/a	0	0	151
3	15	1	n/a	0	0	151
3	15	1	n/a	0	0	151
2	12	2	1	1	0	67
2	13	1	1	5	1	174
1	8	0	1	3	0	184
1	16	0	n/a	3	1	91
4	15	3	n/a	1	0	75
3	16	1	1	1	0	184
3	17	1	0	0	0	161
3	18	2	0	1	0	170
2	13	2	0	1	0	190
2	14	1	1	1	0	101
3	15	2	1	1	0	211
3	12	2	3	1	0	127

BREADS AND CRACKERS

FOOD ITEM	SERVING SIZE	CALORIES
Bread, white	1 slice (approx. 1 oz)	66
Bread, white, reduced-calorie	2 slices (2 oz)	95
Bread, whole-grain	1 slice (approx. 1 oz)	65
Bread, whole-wheat	1 slice (approx. 1 oz)	69
Bread crumbs, dry	1 oz	112
Corn bread	1 oz	89
Cracker, graham	0.75 oz	90
Cracker, melba toast, plain	0.75 oz	83
Cracker, melba toast, rye	0.75 oz	83
Cracker, melba toast, wheat	0.75 oz	80
Cracker, saltine	0.75 oz	91
Cracker, saltine, fat-free	0.75 oz	84
Cracker, Wheat Thins	31 g	147
Croissant	½ medium	116
Croissant, cheese	½ medium	118
English muffin	½ (1 oz)	67
English muffin, cinnamon-raisin	½ (1 oz)	68
English muffin, whole-wheat	½ (1 oz)	67
French toast	½ slice (1 oz)	74
Muffin, blueberry	½ (1 oz)	111
Muffin, bran	½ (1 oz)	77
Muffin, plain, low-fat	½ (1 oz)	84
Muffin, wheat bran	½ (1 oz)	53
Pancake, blueberry	½ of 6 in. pancake (1 oz)	85

PROTEIN (G)	CARB (G)	FIBER (G)	SUGAR (G)	FAT (G)	SAT FAT (G)	SODIUM (MG)
2	13	1	1	1	0	170
4	20	4	2	1	0	208
3	12	2	3	1	0	127
4	12	2	2	1	0	132
4	20	1	2	2	0	208
2	14	1	n/a	3	1	221
1	16	1	7	2	0	129
3	16	1	0	1	0	177
2	16	2	n/a	1	0	191
3	16	2	n/a	0	0	178
2	15	1	0	2	0	228
2	18	1	0	0	0	135
3	20	1	4	6	1.5	246
2	13	1	3	6	3	212
3	13	1	3	6	3	158
2	13	1	1	1	0	132
2	14	1	4	1	0	95
3	13	2	3	1	0	156
3	8	0	n/a	4	1	156
2	14	1	8	5	1	89
2	14	1	3	2	0	111
2	12	1	11	3	1	133
1	10	1	3	2	0	89
2	11	0	n/a	4	1	159

BREADS AND CRACKERS

FOOD ITEM	SERVING SIZE	CALORIES
Pancake, buckwheat	½ of 5 in. pancake (1 oz)	57
Pancake, buttermilk	1 (4 in.) pancake (1 oz)	64
Pancake, plain	1 (4 in.) pancake (1 oz)	64
Pancake, whole-wheat	½ of 5 in. pancake (1 oz)	53
Roll, dinner, plain	1 (1 oz)	87
Roll, dinner, whole-wheat	1 (1 oz)	74
Roll, French	1 (over 1 oz)	105
Roll, hamburger bun	½ (less than 1 oz)	60
Roll, hot dog bun	½ (1 oz)	60
Roll, kaiser	½ (less than 1 oz)	84
Taco shell, baked	1 (0.5 oz)	59
Tortilla, flour	1 (10 in.)	225
Tortilla, wheat	1 (11 in.)	207
Waffle, plain	½ (1 oz)	82

CEREALS

FOOD ITEM	SERVING SIZE	CALORIES
All-Bran	½ c	80
Basic 4	¼ c	52
Bran flakes with raisins, Post Raisin Bran	⅓ c	62
Cheerios	½ c	55
Cheerios, Honey Nut	½ c	56
Cheerios, MultiGrain	½ c	57
Corn Flakes	½ c	50

PROTEIN (G)	CARB (G)	FIBER (G)	SUGAR (G)	FAT (G)	SAT FAT (G)	SODIUM (MG)
2	11	1	1	1	0	168
2	11	1	3	1.5	0	143
2	18	0	n/a	3	1	124
2	10	1	1	0.5	0	113
3	15	1	2	2	0	150
2	14	2	2	1	0	134
3	19	1	0	2	0	231
2	11	1	1	1	0	103
2	11	1	1	1	0	103
3	15	1	1	1	0	155
1	8	1	0	3	1	49
6	37	2	1	6	1	458
8	56	5	n/a	1	0	485
2	9	1	1	4	1	145

PROTEIN (G)	CARB (G)	FIBER (G)	SUGAR (G)	FAT (G)	SAT FAT (G)	SODIUM (MG)
4	23	10	6	1	0	80
1	11	1	4	1	0	80
2	15	2	5	0	0	95
2	11	1	1	1	0	105
1	12	1	5	1	0	135
1	13	1	3	1	0	104
1	12	1	1	0	0	133

CEREALS

FOOD ITEM	SERVING SIZE	CALORIES
Cracklin' Oat Bran	¼ c	67
Cream of Rice, cooked	½ c	63
Cream of Rice, uncooked	2 Tbsp	75
Fiber One	½ c	60
Granola, homemade	¼ c	149
Grape-Nuts	¼ c	104
Grape-Nuts Flakes	½ c	70
Kashi 7 Whole Grain Nuggets	½ c	210
Kashi 7 Whole Grain Puffs	1 c	70
Kashi GOLEAN	½ c	70
Muesli, dried fruit and nuts	¼ c	72
Multigrain hot cereal	½ c	101
Multigrain oatmeal	½ c	71
Oat bran	¼ c	58
Oat bran flakes	⅓ c	47
Oatmeal Crisp, Hearty Raisin	⅓ c	69
100% Bran	⅓ c	83
Raisin Bran	⅓ c	63
Raisin Bran Crunch	⅓ c	63
Rice Krispies	½ c	54
Shredded wheat cereal	1 single-serve box (1 oz)	96
Special K	½ c	60
Steel cut oats, organic, uncooked	2 Tbsp	74
Total	½ c	66
Total Raisin Bran	⅓ c	57
Wheaties	½ c	55

PROTEIN (G)	CARB (G)	FIBER (G)	SUGAR (G)	FAT (G)	SAT FAT (G)	SODIUM (MG)
1	12	2	5	2	1	50
1	14	0	0	0	0	211
1	17	0	0	0	0	1
2	25	14	0	1	0	105
5	16	3	6	7	1	8
3	24	3	3	1	0	177
2	16	2	3	1	0	92
7	47	7	3	2	0	260
2	15	1	0	1	0	0
7	15	5	3	1	0	43
2	17	2	7	1	0	49
3	20	2	1	1	0	1
2	16	3	0	1	0	4
4	16	4	0	2	0	1
2	8	1	1	1	0	27
2	15	1	6	1	0	73
4	23	8	7	1	0	121
2	15	2	6	0	0	117
1	15	1	7	0	0	70
1	12	0	1	0	0	133
3	22	3	0	0.5	0	2
4	11	0	2	0	0	110
3	14	2	0	1	0	1
1	15	2	3	0	0	125
1	14	2	6	0	0	80
2	12	2	2	0	0	105

CHEESE

FOOD ITEM	SERVING SIZE	CALORIES
American, pasteurized process, fat-free	1 in. cube	24
American, pasteurized process, low-fat	1 in. cube	32
American, pasteurized process, low-sodium	1 in. cube	68
American cheese food	1 oz	93
American cheese food, low-fat	1 in. cube	32
Blue, crumbled	1 Tbsp	30
Brie	1 in. cube	57
Cheddar	1 in. cube	69
Cheddar, fat-free	1 in. cube	40
Cheddar, low-fat	1 in. cube	30
Cottage cheese, low-fat 1%	4 oz	81
Cottage cheese, fat-free, large curd, dry	½ c	96
Cottage cheese, low-fat 2%	¼ c	51
Cream cheese	2 Tbsp	101
Cream cheese, fat-free	2 Tbsp	28
Cream cheese, low-fat	2 Tbsp	69
Feta	1 in. cube	45
Gouda	1 oz	101
Monterey Jack, fat-free	1 in. cube	40
Monterey Jack, low-fat	1 in. cube	53
Mozzarella, fat-free, shredded	¼ oz	42
Mozzarella, low-sodium	1 in. cube	50
Mozzarella, part-skim, low moisture	1 oz	86
Mozzarella, string	1 (1 oz)	80

PROTEIN (G)	CARB (G)	FIBER (G)	SUGAR (G)	FAT (G)	SAT FAT (G)	SODIUM (MG)
4	2	0	2	0	0	244
4	1	0	0	1	1	257
4	0	0	0	6	4	1
6	2	0	2	7	4	452
4	1	0	0	1	1	257
2	0	0	0	2.5	1.5	118
4	0	0	0	5	3	107
4	0	0	0	6	4	106
8	1	0	1	0	0	220
4	0	0	0	1	1	106
14	3	0	3	1	1	459
20	2	0	2	0	0	15
8	2	0	0	1	1	229
2	1	0	0	10	6	86
4	2	0	0	0.5	0	158
3	2	0	0	5	3	89
2	1	0	1	4	3	190
7	1	0	1	8	5	232
8	1	0	1	0	0	220
5	0	0	0	4	2	96
9	1	1	0	0	0	210
5	1	0	0	3	2	3
7	1	0	0	6	4	150
8	1	0	0	6	3	240

CHEESE

FOOD ITEM	SERVING SIZE	CALORIES
Muenster	1 in. cube	66
Muenster, low-fat	1 in. cube	49
Parmesan, grated	2 Tbsp	43
Parmesan, hard	1 in. cube	40
Provolone	1 in. cube	60
Ricotta	¼ c	107
Ricotta, low-fat	¼ c	85
Swiss	1 in. cube	57
Swiss, low-fat	1 in. cube	27
Swiss, low-fat, singles	1 slice	50

CONDIMENTS, DRESSINGS, MARINADES, AND SPREADS

FOOD ITEM	SERVING SIZE	CALORIES
Barbecue sauce	1 Tbsp	26
Cocktail sauce, Steel's Gourmet, no sugar added	4 Tbsp	30
Dressing, bacon and tomato	1 Tbsp	49
Dressing, balsamic vinegar	1 Tbsp	14
Dressing, blue cheese	1 Tbsp	76
Dressing, blue cheese, fat-free	1 Tbsp	20
Dressing, blue cheese, low-calorie	1 Tbsp	15
Dressing, Caesar	1 Tbsp	78
Dressing, Caesar, low-fat	1 Tbsp	16
Dressing, Catalina, fat-free	1 Tbsp	18
Dressing, creamy Italian, fat-free	1 Tbsp	25

PROTEIN (G)	CARB (G)	FIBER (G)	SUGAR (G)	FAT (G)	SAT FAT (G)	SODIUM (MG)
4	0	0	0	5	3	113
4	1	0	1	3	2	108
4	0	0	0	3	2	153
4	0	0	0	3	2	165
4	0	0	0	5	3	149
7	2	0	0	8	5	52
7	3	0	0	5	3	77
4	1	0	0	4	3	29
4	1	0	0	1	1	39
8	1	0	0	1	1	73

PROTEIN (G)	CARB (G)	FIBER (G)	SUGAR (G)	FAT (G)	SAT FAT (G)	SODIUM (MG)
0	6	0	5	0	0	196
2	5	0	3	0	0	220
0	0	0	0	5	1	163
0	3	0	2	0	0	4
1	1	0	1	8	1	164
0	4	1	2	0	0	136
1	0	0	0	1	0	180
0	0	0	0	8	1	158
0	3	0	2	1	0	162
0	4	1	4	0	0	160
0	6	0	3	0	0	165

CONDIMENTS, DRESSINGS, MARINADES, AND SPREADS

FOOD ITEM	SERVING SIZE	CALORIES
Dressing, French	1 Tbsp	73
Dressing, French, fat-free	1 Tbsp	21
Dressing, French, reduced-calorie	1 Tbsp	32
Dressing, honey Dijon, low-fat	1 Tbsp	18
Dressing, honey mustard	1 Tbsp	51
Dressing, Italian, reduced fat, without salt	1 Tbsp	11
Dressing, Italian, fat-free	1 Tbsp	7
Dressing, Italian, Kraft Light Done Right!	1 Tbsp	26
Dressing, Italian, reduced-calorie	1 Tbsp	28
Dressing, ranch	1 Tbsp	73
Dressing, ranch, fat-free	1 Tbsp	17
Dressing, ranch, low-fat	1 Tbsp	23
Dressing, ranch, reduced-fat	1 Tbsp	33
Dressing, red wine vinaigrette, fat-free	1 Tbsp	8
Dressing, Russian, low-calorie	1 Tbsp	23
Dressing, Thousand Island	1 Tbsp	59
Dressing, Thousand Island, fat-free	1 Tbsp	21
Dressing, Thousand Island, reduced-fat	1 Tbsp	31
Horseradish	1 Tbsp	7
Horseradish sauce	1 Tbsp	30
Ketchup	1 Tbsp	15
Mustard	1 Tbsp	10
Olives	5 small	18
Olives	5 large	25

PROTEIN (G)	CARB (G)	FIBER (G)	SUGAR (G)	FAT (G)	SAT FAT (G)	SODIUM (MG)
0	2	0	3	7	1	134
0	5	0	3	0	0	128
0	4	0	4	2	0	160
0	2	0	2	1	0	100
0	7	0	7	3	0	37
0	1	0	1	1	0	4
0	1	0	1	0	0	158
0	1	0	1	2	0	114
0	1	0	0	3	0	199
0	1	0	0	8	n/a	122
0	4	0	1	0	0	106
0	4	0	2	1	0	165
0	2	0	0	3	0	140
0	2	0	2	0	0	200
0	4	0	4	1	0	139
0	2	0	2	6	1	138
0	5	1	3	0	0	117
0	3	0	3	2	0	125
0	2	0	1	0	0	47
0	1	0	n/a	3	2	10
0	4	0	3	0	0	167
1	1	1	0	1	0	170
0	1	1	0	2	0	140
0	1	1	0	2	0	192

CONDIMENTS, DRESSINGS, MARINADES, AND SPREADS

FOOD ITEM	SERVING SIZE	CALORIES
Olives	5 jumbo	34
Olives	5 super colossal	62
Pickle, dill	1 small	4
Pickle, dill	1 medium	8
Pickle, dill	1 large	16
Salsa	1 Tbsp	4
Soy sauce	1 Tbsp	11
Soy sauce, low-sodium	1 Tbsp	10
Tabasco sauce	1 Tbsp	2
Tahini	1 Tbsp	89
Vinaigrette, balsamic	1 Tbsp	45
Vinaigrette, red wine	1 Tbsp	45
Wasabi	1 Tbsp	9
Worcestershire sauce	1 Tbsp	11

DAIRY PRODUCTS (*ALSO SEE* CHEESE)

FOOD ITEM	SERVING SIZE	CALORIES
Milk, fat-free	1 c	86
Milk, 1%	1 c	102
Milk, 2%	1 c	122
Milk, whole	1 c	146
Sour cream	1 Tbsp	31
Yogurt, banana, low-fat	4 oz	120
Yogurt, blueberry–French vanilla, low-fat	4 oz	120
Yogurt, coffee, fat-free	4 oz	103
Yogurt, plain, whole milk	4 oz	69

PROTEIN (G)	CARB (G)	FIBER (G)	SUGAR (G)	FAT (G)	SAT FAT (G)	SODIUM (MG)
0	2	1	0	3	0	373
1	4	2	0	5	1	682
0	1	0	0	0	0	324
0	2	1	1	0	0	569
1	4	2	2	0	0	1,181
0	1	0	0	0	0	96
2	1	0	0	0	0	1,005
1	2	0	0	0	0	533
0	0	0	n/a	0	0	89
3	3	1	n/a	8	1	5
0	2	0	2	4	1.5	150
0	1	0	12	5	0	240
0	2	1	0	0	0	1
0	3	0	2	0	0	167

PROTEIN (G)	CARB (G)	FIBER (G)	SUGAR (G)	FAT (G)	SAT FAT (G)	SODIUM (MG)
8	12	0	12	0	0	127
8	12	0	13	2	2	107
8	11	0	12	5	3	100
8	11	0	12	8	5	98
0	1	0	0	3	2	8
5	21	0	18	2	2	60
5	24	0	21	1	0	70
6	20	0	20	0	0	78
4	5	0	5	4	2	52

DAIRY PRODUCTS (*ALSO SEE* CHEESE)

FOOD ITEM	SERVING SIZE	CALORIES
Yogurt, plain, skim milk	4 oz	63
Yogurt, plain, low-fat	4 oz	71
Yogurt, strawberry, fat-free, Breyer's	4 oz	62
Yogurt, strawberry, low-fat, Breyer's	4 oz	109
Yogurt, vanilla, low-fat	4 oz	96

DESSERTS AND SWEET TREATS

FOOD ITEM	SERVING SIZE	CALORIES
Brownie, prepared from recipe	2 in. square	112
Cake, German chocolate	1 slice (2¾ oz)	280
Cake, yellow, with chocolate frosting	1 piece (⅛ of 18 oz cake)	243
Candy, Almond Joy	1 fun size	91
Candy, chocolate bar with almonds	1 fun size (nugget)	60
Candy, chocolate-covered almond	1 (½ oz)	100
Candy, hard, sugar-free	1 piece	11
Candy, M&M'S Peanut	1 fun size	93
Candy, M&M'S Plain	1 fun size	89
Candy, milk chocolate bar	1 mini bar (0.25 oz)	37
Candy, Tootsie Pop	1	26
Candy, Twix	1 oz	143
Cheesecake	1 piece (¹⁄₁₂ of 9 in. cake)	271
Cookie, butter, commercially prepared	0.5 oz	66

PROTEIN (G)	CARB (G)	FIBER (G)	SUGAR (G)	FAT (G)	SAT FAT (G)	SODIUM (MG)
6	9	0	9	0	0	87
6	8	0	8	2	1	79
4	11	0	9	0	0	51
4	21	0	20	1	1	59
6	16	0	16	1	1	75

PROTEIN (G)	CARB (G)	FIBER (G)	SUGAR (G)	FAT (G)	SAT FAT (G)	SODIUM (MG)
1	12	n/a	n/a	7	2	82
3	35	0	24	15	5	300
2	35	1	n/a	11	3	216
1	11	1	9	5	3	27
1	5	0	4	4	2	5
2	9	0	7	6	3	10
0	3	0	0	0	0	0
2	11	1	9	5	2	9
1	13	1	11	4	2	11
1	4	0	4	2	1	6
0	6	0	4	0	0	3
1	19	0	14	7	5	56
5	35	2	21	13	7	376
1	10	0	3	3	2	5

DESSERTS AND SWEET TREATS

FOOD ITEM	SERVING SIZE	CALORIES
Cookie, chocolate chip	0.5 oz	70
Cookie, fig bar	1	56
Cookie, fortune	1	30
Cookie, fudge and caramel	1 small	80
Cookie, oatmeal	1	81
Cookie, oatmeal raisin	1	65
Cookie, sugar	1	72
Doughnut, cake, chocolate	1 (3 in. dia)	175
Doughnut, cake, plain	1 (3¼ in dia)	226
Doughnut hole, cake, plain	1	59
Frozen yogurt, chocolate	½ c	110
Frozen yogurt, chocolate, fat-free	½ c	100
Frozen yogurt, coffee	½ c	110
Frozen yogurt, vanilla, soft serve	½ c	117
Frozen yogurt, vanilla, low-fat	½ c	160
Gum, chewing, regular	1 stick	7
Ice cream, chocolate	½ c	143
Ice cream, chocolate, 98% fat-free, Breyer's	½ c	92
Ice cream, chocolate, sugar-free	½ c	109
Ice cream, vanilla	½ c	145
Ice cream, vanilla, low-fat, Breyer's All Natural Light	½ c	110
Ice cream, vanilla, sugar-free, Breyer's	½ c	99
Ice cream sandwich	1	144
Pie, apple	1 piece (⅙ of 8 in. pie)	277

PROTEIN (G)	CARB (G)	FIBER (G)	SUGAR (G)	FAT (G)	SAT FAT (G)	SODIUM (MG)
1	10	0	n/a	3	1	33
1	11	1	7	1	0	56
0	7	0	4	0	0	22
1	10	0	7	4	3	15
2	12	1	4	3	1	69
1	11	1	9	2	0	81
1	10	0	6	3	1	54
2	24	1	13	8	2	143
3	25	1	9	3	2	143
1	6	0	2	3	1	78
3	19	1	19	3	2	55
4	18	1	12	1	0	75
3	19	0	19	3	2	55
3	17	0	17	4	2	63
7	33	0	19	0	0	51
0	2	0	2	0	0	0
3	19	1	17	7	4	50
3	21	4	14	1	1	51
3	18	1	4	4	3	54
3	17	1	15	8	5	58
3	17	0	15	3	2	48
3	15	0	4	4	3	46
3	22	1	15	6	3	36
2	40	2	18	13	4	311

DESSERTS AND SWEET TREATS

FOOD ITEM	SERVING SIZE	CALORIES
Pie, banana cream	1 piece (⅛ of 9 in. pie)	387
Pie, blueberry	1 piece (⅙ of 8 in. pie)	271
Pie, Boston cream	1 piece (⅙ of 8 in. pie)	232
Pie, cherry	1 piece (⅙ of 8 in. pie)	304
Pie, pecan, prepared from recipe	1 piece	503
Pie, pumpkin	1 piece (⅛ of 9 in. pie)	316
Sherbet, orange	½ c	107

EGGS

FOOD ITEM	SERVING SIZE	CALORIES
Egg, hard-cooked	1 large	78
Egg, poached	1 large	71
Egg, scrambled	1 large	102
Egg white, cooked	1 large	17
Egg white, Egg Beaters	¼ c	30

ENTRÉES AND SIDE DISHES

FOOD ITEM	SERVING SIZE	CALORIES
Breakfast burrito, ham and cheese	4 oz	210
Burrito, bean	1 piece	224
Burrito, cheese and bean	1 piece	189
Burrito, chicken	8 oz (1 piece)	207
Burrito, meat and bean	1 piece	254

PROTEIN (G)	CARB (G)	FIBER (G)	SUGAR (G)	FAT (G)	SAT FAT (G)	SODIUM (MG)
6	47	1	17	20	5	346
2	41	1	12	12	2	380
2	39	1	33	8	2	132
2	47	1	17	13	3	288
6	64	n/a	n/a	27	5	320
7	41	n/a	n/a	14	5	349
1	23	2	18	1	1	34

PROTEIN (G)	CARB (G)	FIBER (G)	SUGAR (G)	FAT (G)	SAT FAT (G)	SODIUM (MG)
6	1	0	1	5	2	62
6	0	0	0	5	2	147
7	1	0	1	7	2	171
4	0	0	0	0	0	55
6	1	0	0	0	0	115

PROTEIN (G)	CARB (G)	FIBER (G)	SUGAR (G)	FAT (G)	SAT FAT (G)	SODIUM (MG)
9	30	0	2	6	2	500
7	36	n/a	n/a	7	3	493
8	27	n/a	n/a	6	3	583
11	30	2	n/a	5	1	1,756
11	33	n/a	n/a	9	4	668

ENTRÉES AND SIDE DISHES

FOOD ITEM	SERVING SIZE	CALORIES
Chicken, barbecued, breast	3 oz	162
Chicken, barbecued, drumstick	1 (2½ oz)	129
Chicken, buffalo wing, spicy	5 pieces	246
Chicken fajita	8 oz (1 piece)	363
Chicken Parmesan	4 oz	199
Chicken potpie, frozen	1 serving	484
Chili, vegetarian, with beans, canned, Hormel	1 c	205
Chili, with beans, canned	1 c	287
Chili, with beans and turkey, canned, Hormel	1 c	203
Chili, without beans, Hormel	1 c	194
Chili con carne, with beans, canned	½ c	149
Crab cake	1	160
Egg roll	1	107
Enchilada, cheese	1	319
Enchilada, chicken (low calorie)	7 oz	356
Fettuccine Alfredo	8 oz	280
Lasagna, with meat and sauce, low-fat frozen entrée	5 oz	143
Pizza, cheese	1 slice (14 in. pie)	272
Pizza, pepperoni and cheese	1 slice (14 in. pie)	298
Sandwich, chicken salad, on whole-wheat bread	1	398
Sandwich, turkey, on whole-wheat	1	360
Shrimp cocktail	3 oz	81

PROTEIN (G)	CARB (G)	FIBER (G)	SUGAR (G)	FAT (G)	SAT FAT (G)	SODIUM (MG)
20	2	0	n/a	8	2	181
16	2	0	n/a	6	2	145
21	0	0	0	17	5	64
20	44	5	n/a	12	2	343
18	10	1	6	10	3	399
13	43	2	8	29	10	857
12	38	10	6	1	0	778
15	30	11	3	14	6	1,336
19	26	6	6	3	1	1,198
17	18	3	3	7	2	970
9	14	5	n/a	6	2	522
11	5	0	n/a	10	2	491
3	18	1	2	2	1	191
10	29	n/a	n/a	19	11	784
26	29	2	n/a	15	9	1,018
13	40	2	7	7	4	690
10	19	2	n/a	3	1	257
12	34	2	4	10	4	551
13	34	2	4	12	5	683
31	5	3	3	26	3	527
27	29	4	3	16	2.5	1,733
10	8	2	4	1	0	417

ENTRÉES AND SIDE DISHES

FOOD ITEM	SERVING SIZE	CALORIES
Spaghetti and meatballs, canned	½ c	136
Taco, chicken, soft, prepared from recipe	1 (2½ oz)	175

FATS AND OILS

FOOD ITEM	SERVING SIZE	CALORIES
Butter, with salt	1 tsp	34
Butter, without salt	1 tsp	34
Butter-margarine blend, stick, without salt	1 tsp	33
Flaxseed oil	1 tsp	40
Margarine, hard, corn and soybean oils	1 tsp	33
Margarine, hard, corn oil	1 tsp	34
Margarine, hard, soybean oil	1 tsp	34
Margarine, regular, with salt	1 tsp	34
Margarine, regular, without salt	1 tsp	34
Oil, canola	1 tsp	40
Oil, olive	1 tsp	40
Oil, safflower	1 tsp	40
Oil, sesame	1 tsp	40
Oil, walnut	1 tsp	40

FISH

FOOD ITEM	SERVING SIZE	CALORIES
Cod, Atlantic, baked	3 oz	89
Flounder, baked	3 oz	99

PROTEIN (G)	CARB (G)	FIBER (G)	SUGAR (G)	FAT (G)	SAT FAT (G)	SODIUM (MG)
5	14	n/a	4	7	3	518
15	9	1	0.5	8.5	3	134

PROTEIN (G)	CARB (G)	FIBER (G)	SUGAR (G)	FAT (G)	SAT FAT (G)	SODIUM (MG)
0	0	0	0	4	2	27
0	0	0	0	4	2	1
0	0	0	0	4	1	1
0	0	0	0	5	0	0
0	0	0	0	4	1	30
0	0	0	0	4	1	44
0	0	0	0	4	1	44
0	0	0	0	4	1	44
0	0	0	0	4	1	0
0	0	0	0	5	0	0
0	0	0	0	5	1	0
0	0	0	0	5	0	0
0	0	0	0	5	1	0
0	0	0	0	5	0	0

PROTEIN (G)	CARB (G)	FIBER (G)	SUGAR (G)	FAT (G)	SAT FAT (G)	SODIUM (MG)
19	0	0	0	1	0	66
21	0	0	0	1	0	89

FISH

FOOD ITEM	SERVING SIZE	CALORIES
Grouper, baked	3 oz	100
Halibut, Atlantic and Pacific, baked	3 oz	119
Mahi mahi, baked	3 oz	93
Salmon, Alaskan chinook, smoked, canned	3 oz	128
Salmon, pink, canned, drained	3 oz	116
Swordfish, baked	3 oz	132
Tilapia, baked or broiled	3 oz	109
Tuna, bluefin, baked	3 oz	156
Tuna, StarKist Chunk Light, canned in water, drained	2 oz	70
Tuna, white, canned in water, drained	3 oz	109
Tuna, yellowfin, baked	3 oz	118

FRUIT

FOOD ITEM	SERVING SIZE	CALORIES
Apple	1 medium (2¾ in. dia)	72
Apricot	1	17
Avocado	¼ c	58
Banana	1 large (8 in.)	121
Banana	1 extra large (9 in.)	135
Blackberries	1 c	62
Blueberries	½ c	42
Cantaloupe, wedged	⅛ small	19

PROTEIN (G)	CARB (G)	FIBER (G)	SUGAR (G)	FAT (G)	SAT FAT (G)	SODIUM (MG)
21	0	0	0	1	0	45
23	0	0	0	3	0	59
20	0	0	0	1	0	96
20	1	0	0	5	n/a	n/a
20	0	0	0	4	1	339
22	0	0	0	4	1	98
22	0	0	0	2	1	48
25	0	0	0	5	1	42
15	0	0	0	0	0	230
20	0	0	0	3	1	320
25	0	0	0	1	0	40

PROTEIN (G)	CARB (G)	FIBER (G)	SUGAR (G)	FAT (G)	SAT FAT (G)	SODIUM (MG)
0	19	3	14	0	0	1
0	4	1	3	0	0	0
1	3	2	0	5	1	3
1	31	4	17	0	0	1
2	35	4	19	1	0	2
2	14	8	7	1	0	1
1	11	2	7	0	0	1
0	4	1	4	0	0	9

FRUIT

FOOD ITEM	SERVING SIZE	CALORIES
Cantaloupe, wedged	⅛ medium	23
Cantaloupe, wedged	⅛ large	35
Cranberries	1 c	44
Grapefruit, pink, red, white	½ small	32
Grapefruit, pink, red, white	½ medium	41
Grapefruit, pink, red, white	½ large	53
Grapes, green	½ c	52
Grapes, red	½ c	52
Lemon	1 medium (2⅛ in.)	17
Nectarine	1 large (2¾ in.)	69
Orange	1 small (2⅜ in.)	45
Orange	1 large (3 1/16 in.)	86
Peach	1 medium	58
Pear	½ medium	52
Pineapple	¼	57
Plum	1 (2⅛ in.)	30
Raspberries, red	¾ c	48
Strawberry	1 medium	4
Watermelon, sliced	1 wedge (1/16 of melon)	86

GRAINS AND RICES

FOOD ITEM	SERVING SIZE	CALORIES
Couscous, cooked	⅓ c	59
Oat bran, cooked	⅓ c	29

PROTEIN (G)	CARB (G)	FIBER (G)	SUGAR (G)	FAT (G)	SAT FAT (G)	SODIUM (MG)
1	6	1	5	0	0	11
1	8	1	8	0	0	16
0	12	4	4	0	0	2
1	8	1	7	0	0	0
1	10	1	9	0	0	0
1	13	2	12	0	0	0
1	14	1	12	0	0	2
1	14	1	12	0	0	2
1	5	2	1	0	0	1
2	16	3	12	1	0	0
1	11	2	9	0	0	0
2	22	4	17	0	0	0
1	14	2	13	0	0	0
0	14	3	9	0	0	1
1	15	2	11	0	0	1
0	8	1	7	0	0	0
1	11	6	4	1	0	1
0	1	0	1	0	0	2
2	22	1	18	0	0	3

PROTEIN (G)	CARB (G)	FIBER (G)	SUGAR (G)	FAT (G)	SAT FAT (G)	SODIUM (MG)
2	12	1	0	0	0	3
2	8	2	n/a	1	0	1

GRAINS AND RICES

FOOD ITEM	SERVING SIZE	CALORIES
Oats, rolled, dry	2 Tbsp	37
Quinoa, dry	2 Tbsp	79
Rice, brown, long-grain, cooked	¼ c	54
Rice, brown, medium-grain, cooked	¼ c	55
Rice, brown, short-grain, dry	1½ Tbsp	66
Rice, whole-grain, brown, Uncle Ben's 10-minute, dry	¼ c	170
Rice, white, long-grain, cooked	¼ c	51
Rice, wild, cooked	⅓ c	55

MEATS

FOOD ITEM	SERVING SIZE	CALORIES
Beef		
Bottom round, all lean, grilled	3 oz	155
Bottom round, all lean, roasted, boneless	3 oz	144
Bottom round, trimmed, boneless, braised	3 oz	190
Corned beef, cooked	3 oz	213
Corned beef lunchmeat, sliced	3 oz	85
Filet mignon, lean, broiled	3 oz	164
Flank steak, lean, braised	3 oz	201
Flank steak, lean, raw	4 oz	169
Ground patty, 10% fat, raw	4 oz	199

PROTEIN (G)	CARB (G)	FIBER (G)	SUGAR (G)	FAT (G)	SAT FAT (G)	SODIUM (MG)
1	7	1	0	1	0	0
3	15	1	n/a	1	0	4
1	11	1	0	0	0	2
1	11	1	n/a	0	0	0
1	15	1	0	1	0	2
1	35	2	0	1.5	0	0
1	11	0	0	0	0	0
2	12	1	0	0	0	2

PROTEIN (G)	CARB (G)	FIBER (G)	SUGAR (G)	FAT (G)	SAT FAT (G)	SODIUM (MG)
23	0	0	0	6	2	49
24	0	0	0	5	2	32
28	0	0	0	8	3	37
15	0	0	0	16	5	964
13	0	0	0	4	2	982
24	0	0	0	7	3	50
24	0	0	0	11	5	61
25	0	0	0	7	3	65
23	0	0	0	11	5	75

MEATS

FOOD ITEM	SERVING SIZE	CALORIES
Ground, 20% fat, pan broiled	3 oz	209
Ground, 20% fat, raw	4 oz	287
Ground patty, 30% fat, pan broiled	3 oz	202
Ground, 30% fat, raw	4 oz	375
Ground, extra lean, raw (5% fat)	4 oz	155
Hot dog, beef, fat-free	1 frank	62
Roast beef, lunchmeat, medium rare	1 oz	30
Salami, beef, beerwurst	1 oz	78
Salami, beef, cooked	1 oz	74
Sausage, beef, precooked	25 g	101
Steak, top sirloin, ⅛ trim, broiled	3 oz	207
Steak, top sirloin, ⅛ trim, raw	4 oz	228
Steak, top sirloin, lean, broiled	3 oz	160
T-bone, lean, broiled	3 oz	161
T-bone, raw (trimmed to ¼ in. fat)	4 oz	240
Tenderloin, lean, boneless, raw	4 oz	136
Tenderloin, select lean, boneless, roasted	3 oz	139
Pork		
Bacon, medium slice, cooked (fried or roasted)	1 slice	43
Bacon, medium slice, raw	1 slice	157
Canadian bacon, grilled	1 slice	43

PROTEIN (G)	CARB (G)	FIBER (G)	SUGAR (G)	FAT (G)	SAT FAT (G)	SODIUM (MG)
20	0	0	0	14	5	71
19	0	0	0	23	9	76
19	0	0	0	13	5	78
16	0	0	0	34	13	76
24	0	0	0	6	3	75
7	3	0	0	1	0	455
6	1	0	1	1	1	235
4	1	0	0	6	2	205
4	1	0	0	6	3	323
4	0	0	0	19	4	228
23	0	0	0	12	5	48
23	0	0	0	14	6	59
26	0	0	0	6	2	54
22	0	0	0	7	3	60
22	0	0	0	16	6	61
24	0	0	0	4	1	57
24	0	0	0	4	1	48
3	0	0	0	3	1	185
11	0	0	0	12	4	670
6	0	0	0	2	1	363

MEATS

FOOD ITEM	SERVING SIZE	CALORIES
Chop, center lean, with bone, braised	3 oz	172
Chop, with barbecue sauce	4 oz	209
Chop sirloin, lean, raw, boneless	1 chop	129
Chop sirloin, lean, with bone, braised	1 chop	142
Ground, cooked	3 oz	252
Ground, raw	4 oz	297
Ham, low-sodium, 96% fat-free, roasted, boneless	1 oz	47
Ham, rump, lean, raw	4 oz	155
Hot dog, pork	1 link	204
Hotdog, pork, beef, and turkey, fat-free	1 link	50
Meatballs	1 oz (1 meatball)	60
Ribs, country-style, lean, braised	3 oz	199
Ribs, country-style, lean, raw	4 oz	178
Sausage, pork, cooked	1 oz (1 each)	82
Tenderloin, raw, lean	4 oz	136
Tenderloin, roasted, lean	3 oz	139
Tenderloin, teriyaki, Hormel Always Tender	4 oz	133
Tenderloin, lean, broiled	3 oz	159
Veal		
Breast, braised, boneless, lean	3 oz	185
Ground, broiled	3 oz	146
Loin, roasted, lean	3 oz	149

PROTEIN (G)	CARB (G)	FIBER (G)	SUGAR (G)	FAT (G)	SAT FAT (G)	SODIUM (MG)
25	0	0	0	7	3	53
23	3	0	0	11	4	860
21	0	0	0	4	1	52
19	0	0	0	6	2	38
22	0	0	0	18	7	62
19	0	0	0	24	9	63
6	0	0	0	2	1	275
24	0	0	0	6	2	78
10	0	0	0	18	7	620
6	6	0	2	0	0	490
5	2	0	0	3.5	1	35
22	0	0	0	12	4	54
22	0	0	0	9	3	76
4	0	0	0	7.5	3	200
24	0	0	0	4	1	57
24	0	0	0	4	1	48
20	5	n/a	4	3	1	463
26	0	0	n/a	5	2	55
26	0	n/a	n/a	8	3	58
21	0	0	0	6	3	71
22	0	0	0	6	2	82

NUTS, SEEDS, AND BUTTERS

FOOD ITEM	SERVING SIZE	CALORIES
Almond butter, plain, with salt	1 Tbsp	101
Almond butter, plain, without salt	1 Tbsp	101
Almonds, blanched	1 Tbsp	53
Almonds, dry-roasted, blanched	1 Tbsp (¼ oz)	52
Almonds, dry-roasted, with salt	½ oz (11 nuts)	85
Almonds, dry-roasted, without salt	½ oz	85
Almonds, honey-roasted	½ oz	84
Almonds, natural, sliced	½ oz	82
Almonds, oil-roasted, with salt	½ oz	86
Almonds, oil-roasted, without salt	½ oz	86
Brazil nuts, dried	1 nut	33
Brazil nuts, dried	½ oz (3 nuts)	93
Cashew butter, plain, with salt	1 Tbsp	94
Cashew butter, plain, without salt	1 Tbsp	94
Cashew nuts, dry-roasted, with salt	½ oz	81
Cashew nuts, dry-roasted, without salt	1 Tbsp	49
Cashew nuts, raw	½ oz	78
Flaxseeds, ground	1 Tbsp	37
Macadamia nuts, dry-roasted, with salt	½ oz (5–6 nuts)	101
Macadamia nuts, dry-roasted, without salt	½ oz	102
Mixed nuts, dry-roasted, with peanuts, with salt	½ oz	84

PROTEIN (G)	CARB (G)	FIBER (G)	SUGAR (G)	FAT (G)	SAT FAT (G)	SODIUM (MG)
2	3	1	1	9	1	72
2	3	1	n/a	9	1	2
2	2	1	0	5	0	3
2	1	1	0	5	0.5	0
3	3	2	1	7	1	48
3	3	2	1	7	1	0
3	4	2	n/a	7	1	18
3	3	2	1	7	1	0
3	3	2	1	8	1	48
3	3	2	1	8	1	0
1	1	0	0	3	1	0
2	2	1	0	9	2	0
3	4	0	1	8	2	98
3	4	0	1	8	2	2
2	5	0	1	7	1	91
1	3	0	0	4	1	1
3	4	1	1	6	1	2
1	2	2	0	3	0	2
1	2	1	1	11	2	38
1	2	1	1	11	2	1
2	4	1	1	7	1	95

NUTS, SEEDS, AND BUTTERS

FOOD ITEM	SERVING SIZE	CALORIES
Mixed nuts, dry-roasted, with peanuts, without salt	½ oz	84
Mixed nuts, oil-roasted, with peanuts, with salt	½ oz	87
Mixed nuts, oil-roasted, with peanuts, without salt	½ oz	87
Mixed nuts, oil-roasted, without peanuts, with salt	1 Tbsp	87
Mixed nuts, oil-roasted, without peanuts, without salt	½ oz	87
Peanut butter, creamy, with salt	1 Tbsp	94
Peanut butter, creamy, reduced-fat	1 Tbsp	83
Peanut butter, crunchy, with salt	1 Tbsp	94
Peanut butter, natural	1 Tbsp	100
Peanut butter, reduced-sodium	1 Tbsp	101
Peanuts, dry-roasted, with salt	½ oz	83
Peanuts, dry-roasted, without salt	½ oz	83
Peanuts, shelled, cooked, with salt	1 Tbsp	36
Pecans, dried, chopped	⅛ c	94
Pecans, dried, halved	⅛ c	86
Pecans, dry-roasted, with salt	½ oz	101
Pecans, dry-roasted, without salt	½ oz	101
Pecans, oil-roasted, with salt, halved	½ oz	101
Pecans, oil-roasted, without salt, halved	½ oz	101

PROTEIN (G)	CARB (G)	FIBER (G)	SUGAR (G)	FAT (G)	SAT FAT (G)	SODIUM (MG)
2	4	1	1	7	1	2
2	3	1	1	8	1	59
2	3	1	1	8	1	2
2	3	1	1	8	1	43
2	3	1	1	8	1	2
4	3	1	1	8	2	73
4	6	1	1	5	1	86
4	3	1	1	8	1	78
4	4	1	1	8	1	60
4	4	1	1	8	2	32
3	3	1	1	7	1	115
3	3	1	1	7	1	1
2	2	1	0	2.5	0.5	84
1	2	1	1	10	1	0
1	2	1	1	9	1	0
1	2	1	1	11	1	54
1	2	1	1	11	1	0
1	2	1	1	11	1	56
1	2	1	1	11	1	0

NUTS, SEEDS, AND BUTTERS

FOOD ITEM	SERVING SIZE	CALORIES
Pistachios, dry-roasted, with salt	½ oz	81
Pistachios, dry-roasted, without salt	½ oz	81
Walnuts, dried, black	1 Tbsp	48
Walnuts, English, ground	⅛ c	65
Walnuts, dried, halved	½ oz	93

PASTA

FOOD ITEM	SERVING SIZE	CALORIES
Note: For most pasta shapes, 1 ounce of dry pasta makes approximately ½ cup cooked.		
Angel hair, whole-wheat, dry, organic	1 oz	106
Bow-ties, semolina, dry	1 oz	103
Fettuccine (tagliatelle), semolina, dry	1 oz	102
Fettuccine (tagliatelle), spinach, dry	1 oz	98
Lasagna, semolina, dry	1 oz	102
Linguine, semolina, dry	1 oz	102
Penne, semolina, dry	1 oz	106
Penne, whole-wheat, dry, organic	1 oz	106
Spaghetti, brown rice, dry	1 oz	106
Spaghetti, corn, dry	1 oz	101
Spaghetti, semolina, dry, organic	1 oz	102
Spaghetti, spinach, dry, organic	1 oz	106
Spaghetti, whole-wheat, dry, organic	1 oz	99

PROTEIN (G)	CARB (G)	FIBER (G)	SUGAR (G)	FAT (G)	SAT FAT (G)	SODIUM (MG)
3	4	2	1	7	1	57
3	4	2	1	7	1	1
2	1	1	0	5	0	0
2	1	1	0	7	1	0
2	2	1	0	9	1	0

PROTEIN (G)	CARB (G)	FIBER (G)	SUGAR (G)	FAT (G)	SAT FAT (G)	SODIUM (MG)
4	21	3	1	1	0	5
4	21	1	1	0	0	1
4	21	1	1	1	0	2
4	20	1	1	1	0	9
4	21	1	1	1	0	1
4	21	1	1	1	0	2
4	22	1	1	0.5	0	3
4	21	3	1	1	0	5
2	21	1	0	0	0	n/a
2	22	3	n/a	1	0	1
4	21	1	1	1	0	3
4	21	3	0	0.5	0	10
4	21	4	1	0.5	0	2

POULTRY

FOOD ITEM	SERVING SIZE	CALORIES
Chicken		
Chicken, breast, boneless, without skin, stewed	½ breast	143
Chicken, breast, boneless, without skin, raw	½ breast	128
Chicken, breast, oven-roasted, fat-free, sliced, Oscar Mayer	6 slices	66
Chicken, breast, with bone, with skin, raw	½ breast	249
Chicken, breast, with bone, with skin, roasted	1 lb	114
Chicken, drumstick, with skin, cooked	1 drumstick	112
Chicken, drumstick, with skin, raw	1 drumstick	118
Chicken, drumstick, without skin, roasted	1 drumstick	76
Chicken, drumstick, without skin, raw	1 drumstick	74
Chicken, thigh, boneless, without skin, roasted	1 thigh	109
Chicken, thigh, boneless, without skin, raw	1 thigh	82
Chicken, thigh, with bone, with skin, raw	1 thigh	198
Chicken, thigh, with bone, with skin, roasted	1 thigh	153
Chicken frankfurter	1	116
Chicken lunchmeat, deli	1 oz	23
Turkey		
Turkey, breast, fat-free, smoked, Oscar Mayer	3 slices	31
Turkey, breast, raw, with skin	from 1 lb turkey	154
Turkey, breast, with skin, roasted	from 1 lb turkey	150

PROTEIN (G)	CARB (G)	FIBER (G)	SUGAR (G)	FAT (G)	SAT FAT (G)	SODIUM (MG)
23	0	0	0	3	1	77
27	0	0	0	1	0	60
14	1	0	1	0	0	969
30	0	0	0	13	4	91
17	0	0	0	5	1	41
14	0	0	0	6	2	47
14	0	0	0	6	2	61
12	0	0	0	2	1	42
13	0	0	0	2	1	55
13	0	0	0	6	2	46
14	0	0	0	3	1	59
16	0	0	0	14	4	71
16	0	0	0	10	3	52
6	3	0	0	9	2	616
5	0	0	0	0	0	210
6	1	0	0	0	0	427
29	0	0	0	3	1	59
28	0	0	0	3	1	52

POULTRY

FOOD ITEM	SERVING SIZE	CALORIES
Turkey, dark meat, with skin, roasted	from 1 lb turkey	230
Turkey, dark meat, without skin, roasted	from 1 lb turkey	147
Turkey, drumstick, with skin, smoked	3 oz	131
Turkey, drumstick, without skin, cooked	3 oz	159
Turkey, ground, cooked	3 oz	145
Turkey, leg, with skin, raw	from 1 lb turkey	151
Turkey, leg, with skin, roasted	from 1 lb turkey	148
Turkey, light meat, with skin, roasted	frm ½ lb turkey	134
Turkey, light meat, with skin, smoked	3 oz	177
Turkey, light meat, without skin, roasted	from 1 lb turkey	146
Turkey, light meat, without skin, smoked	2 thick slices	143
Turkey, wing, with skin, smoked	3 oz	131
Turkey frankfurter	1	102
Turkey sausage, smoked, hot	1 oz	44

SEAFOOD

FOOD ITEM	SERVING SIZE	CALORIES
Crab, Alaskan, king crab, steamed	3 oz	82
Crab, baked or broiled	3 oz	117
Crab, imitation (surimi)	3 oz	81
Crab, sautéed	3 oz	117
Lobster, Northern, steamed	3 oz	83

PROTEIN (G)	CARB (G)	FIBER (G)	SUGAR (G)	FAT (G)	SAT FAT (G)	SODIUM (MG)
29	0	0	0	12	4	79
26	0	0	0	4	1	72
18	0	0	0	6	2	627
24	0	0	0	6	2	67
17	0	0	0	8	2	66
21	0	0	0	7	2	78
20	0	0	0	7	2	55
19	0	0	0	6	2	43
24	0	0	0	8	2	847
31	0	0	n/a	1	0	58
25	0	0	0	4	1	837
16	0	0	0	7	2	568
6	1	0	0	8	3	642
4	1	0	1	2	1	260

PROTEIN (G)	CARB (G)	FIBER (G)	SUGAR (G)	FAT (G)	SAT FAT (G)	SODIUM (MG)
16	0	0	0	1	0	911
16	0	0	n/a	5.5	1	270
6	13	0	5	0	0	715
16	0	0	0	5	1	270
17	1	0	0	1	0	323

SEAFOOD

FOOD ITEM	SERVING SIZE	CALORIES
Shrimp, cooked	3 oz	84
Shrimp, steamed	1 large	5

SNACKS

FOOD ITEM	SERVING SIZE	CALORIES
Baked! Cheetos Crunchy Cheese Flavored Snacks	1 oz	130
Baked! Doritos Nacho Cheese	1 oz	120
Baked! Lay's Cheddar & Sour Cream Flavored Potato Crisps	1 oz	120
Baked! Lay's Original Potato Crisps	1 oz	110
Baked! Tostitos Original Bite Size	1 oz	110
Chex Party Mix	1 oz	120
Corn chips	1 oz	147
Granola bar, almond, hard	1	119
Granola bar, chocolate chip, hard	1	105
Jerky, beef	1 oz	116
Popcorn, air-popped	1 c	31
Popcorn, microwaveable, low-fat, low-sodium	0.5 oz	60
Popcorn, microwaveable, 94% fat-free	0.5 oz	57
Potato chips, baked	1 c	159
Potato chips, fat-free	0.5 oz	54
Potato chips, light	0.5 oz	71
Potato chips, reduced-fat	0.5 oz	68

PROTEIN (G)	CARB (G)	FIBER (G)	SUGAR (G)	FAT (G)	SAT FAT (G)	SODIUM (MG)
17	0	0	0	1	0	190
1	0	0	0	0	0	12

PROTEIN (G)	CARB (G)	FIBER (G)	SUGAR (G)	FAT (G)	SAT FAT (G)	SODIUM (MG)
2	19	0	1	5	1	240
2	21	2	1	4	1	220
2	21	2	3	4	1	210
2	23	2	2	2	0	150
3	24	2	0	1	0	200
3	18	2	n/a	5	2	288
2	18	0	n/a	8	6	290
2	15	1	n/a	6	3	61
2	17	1	n/a	4	3	83
9	3	1	3	7	3	627
1	6	1	0	0	0	1
2	10	2	0	1	0	69
1	11	2	0	1	0	89
2	24	2	2	6	1	312
1	12	1	1	0	0	91
1	9	1	1	4	1	61
1	9	1	0	3	1	70

SNACKS

FOOD ITEM	SERVING SIZE	CALORIES
Potato chips, reduced-fat, unsalted	0.5 oz	69
Pretzel, hard	1	23
Pretzel, hard, twist, unsalted	1	23
Pretzel, hard, whole-wheat	0.5 oz	51
Pretzel, soft	1 medium	389
Tortilla chips, baked, light	10 chips	74
Tortilla chips, baked, low-fat	0.5 oz	59
Tortilla chips, baked, without salt	10 chips	66
Trail mix	0.5 oz	65

SOUPS, SAUCES, AND GRAVIES

FOOD ITEM	SERVING SIZE	CALORIES
Gravy, au jus, canned	2 Tbsp	2
Gravy, beef, canned	1 Tbsp	8
Sauce, Alfredo	2 Tbsp	55
Sauce, barbecue	2 Tbsp	52
Sauce, enchilada, Ortega	1 Tbsp	8
Sauce, marinara	1 Tbsp	12
Sauce, pasta, with meat, Prego	1 Tbsp	18
Sauce, sweet-and-sour, Nestlé	1 Tbsp	25
Sauce, taco, red, La Victoria	1 Tbsp	7
Sauce, tamari	1 Tbsp	11
Sauce, teriyaki	1 Tbsp	15
Sauce, tomato, with salt	½ c	29
Sauce, tomato, without salt, canned	½ c	45

PROTEIN (G)	CARB (G)	FIBER (G)	SUGAR (G)	FAT (G)	SAT FAT (G)	SODIUM (MG)
1	9	1	0	3	1	1
1	5	0	n/a	0	0	81
1	5	0	n/a	0	0	17
2	12	1	n/a	0	0	29
9	80	2	0	4	1	1,615
1	12	1	0	2	0	160
2	11	1	0	1	0	59
2	13	1	0	1	0	67
2	6	n/a	n/a	4	1	32

PROTEIN (G)	CARB (G)	FIBER (G)	SUGAR (G)	FAT (G)	SAT FAT (G)	SODIUM (MG)
0	1	0	n/a	0	0	7
1	1	0	0	1	0	82
1	1	0	0	5	2	195
0	13	0	9	0	0	392
0	1	0	0	0	0	39
0	2	0	1	0	0	75
0	3	0	2	1	0	66
0	6	0	4	0	0	115
0	1	0	1	0	0	105
2	1	0	0	0	0	1,005
1	3	0	2	0	0	670
2	7	2	5	0	0	642
2	9	2	5	0	0	13

SOUPS, SAUCES, AND GRAVIES

FOOD ITEM	SERVING SIZE	CALORIES
Soup, bean and bacon	1 c	106
Soup, beef and vegetable	1 c	78
Soup, black bean	½ c	58
Soup, chicken noodle	1 c	75
Soup, chicken noodle, chunky, canned	1 c	175
Soup, chicken noodle, low-sodium	1 c	76
Soup, chili, beef	1 c	170
Soup, clam chowder, Manhattan-style	1 c	78
Soup, clam chowder, New England–style	1 c	95
Soup, crab, canned	1 c	76
Soup, cream of mushroom	1 c	96
Soup, French onion, Campbell's, prepared	1 c	90
Soup, gazpacho, canned	1 c	46
Soup, green pea	1 c	165
Soup, lentil, fat-free, canned	½ c	55
Soup, minestrone	1 c	82
Soup, tomato	1 c	85
Soup, vegetable	1 c	75

VEGETABLES

FOOD ITEM	SERVING SIZE	CALORIES
Alfalfa sprouts	½ c	4
Artichoke	1 medium	60
Asparagus, cooked	8 spears	26

PROTEIN (G)	CARB (G)	FIBER (G)	SUGAR (G)	FAT (G)	SAT FAT (G)	SODIUM (MG)
5	16	9	1	2	1	928
6	10	1	1	2	1	791
3	10	2	1	1	0	599
4	9	1	0	2	1	1,106
13	17	4	2	6	1	850
4	11	1	0	2	1	426
7	21	10	7	7	3	1,035
2	12	2	1	2	0	578
5	12	2	0	3	0	915
5	10	1	n/a	2	0	1,235
2	8	0	2	7	2	731
4	12	2	8	3	1	1,800
7	4	1	1	0	0	739
9	27	5	8	3	1	918
5	13	5	4	0	0	225
4	11	1	n/a	3	1	911
2	17	1	9	2	0	695
4	9	1	1	3	1	945

PROTEIN (G)	CARB (G)	FIBER (G)	SUGAR (G)	FAT (G)	SAT FAT (G)	SODIUM (MG)
1	0	0	0	0	0	1
4	13	7	1	0	0	397
3	5	2	2	0	0	17

VEGETABLES

FOOD ITEM	SERVING SIZE	CALORIES
Bell pepper, chopped	1 c	30
Bell pepper, boiled	1 c	38
Broccoli, chopped, boiled	1 c	55
Broccoli, florets, fresh	1 c	20
Brussels sprouts, raw	1 c	38
Cabbage, raw	1 medium leaf	6
Carrot	1 medium	25
Carrot, baby	1 medium	4
Cauliflower	¼ medium head	36
Celery	1 medium stalk	6
Celery, chopped	1 c	16
Cherry tomatoes, red	1 c	27
Corn, sweet white	½ c	66
Corn, sweet white	1 small ear	63
Corn, sweet white	1 large ear	123
Corn, sweet yellow	½ c	66
Corn, sweet yellow	1 small ear	63
Corn, sweet yellow	1 large ear	123
Cucumber with peel, raw	1 (8¼ in.)	45
Garlic	1 clove	4
Green beans, snap, raw	1 c	34
Green beans, with almonds, frozen, Green Giant	1 c	91
Lettuce, iceberg	5 large leaves	10
Lettuce, romaine	4 leaves	19
Mushrooms, brown Italian	5	27
Onion, green (scallions), tops and bulbs, chopped	½ c	16

PROTEIN (G)	CARB (G)	FIBER (G)	SUGAR (G)	FAT (G)	SAT FAT (G)	SODIUM (MG)
1	7	3	4	0	0	4
1	9	2	3	0	0	3
4	11	5	2	1	0	64
2	4	2	0	0	0	19
3	8	3	2	0	0	22
0	1	1	1	0	0	4
1	6	2	3	0	0	42
0	1	0	0	0	0	8
3	8	4	3	0	0	43
0	1	1	1	0	0	32
1	3	2	2	0	0	81
1	6	2	4	0	0	7
2	15	2	2	1	0	12
2	14	2	2	1	0	11
5	27	4	5	2	0	21
2	15	2	2	1	0	12
2	14	2	2	1	0	11
5	27	4	5	2	0	21
2	11	2	5	0	0	6
0	1	0	0	0	0	1
2	8	4	2	0	0	7
3	8	3	3	4.5	0	144
1	2	1	1	0	0	8
1	4	2	1	0	0	9
3	4	1	2	0	0	6
1	4	1	1	0	0	8

VEGETABLES

FOOD ITEM	SERVING SIZE	CALORIES
Onion, red	1 medium	44
Onion, yellow	1 medium	44
Peas, green, raw	½ c	59
Peas, snow, whole, raw	½ c	13
Potato, baked, with skin, without salt	1 medium	161
Sauerkraut, canned, low-sodium	1 c	31
Snap beans, green	1 c	27
Spinach	3 oz	20
Spinach, baby, Dole	1 c	10
Spinach, cooked, with salt	1 c	41
Spinach, cooked, without salt	1 c	41
Squash, summer	1 medium	31
Sweet potato, baked, with skin, without salt	1 small	54
Sweet potato, baked, without skin, without salt	1 medium	103
Tomato, red	1 medium	22
Zucchini, with skin, raw	1 medium	31

PROTEIN (G)	CARB (G)	FIBER (G)	SUGAR (G)	FAT (G)	SAT FAT (G)	SODIUM (MG)
1	10	2	5	0	0	4
1	10	2	5	0	0	4
4	10	4	4	0	0	4
1	2	1	1	0	0	1
4	37	4	2	0	0	17
1	6	4	3	0	0	437
1	7	4	3	0	0	0
2	3	2	0	0	0	67
1	3	1	0	0	0	39
5	7	4	1	0	0	551
5	7	4	1	0	0	126
2	7	2	4	0	0	4
1	12	2	4	0	0	22
2	24	4	10	0	0	41
1	5	1	3	0	0	6
2	7	2	3	0	0	20

Index

Underscored page references indicate tables and sidebars. **Boldface** references indicate photographs.

Subway, best and worst meals from, 118
Sucralose, 57
Sugar alcohols, 58
Sugar substitutes, 57–58
Sunflower seeds, nutrients in, 92–93
Sushi, best and worst, 128–29
Sweet'n Low, 57
Sweet potato, nutrients in, 76–77
Sweets, satisfying cravings for, 33, 47, 56
Swiss ball pushup, 152, **152**
Swiss chard
  nutrients in, 47, 82–83
  preparing, 47

Taco Bell, best and worst meals from, 118–19
Tahini, nutrients in, 82–83
Tea
  caffeine in, 53
  green
    for bad breath, 61–62
    for boosting metabolism, 24
    nutrients in, 78–79
  for weight loss, 46
Teeth cleaners, foods as, 65
Thermic effect of food, metabolism and, 19, 22
Tomatoes, nutrients in, 74–75
Tonic water, for calf cramps, 63
Tootsie Pop, 56
Trail mix, 34
Trout, nutrients in, 84–85
Tuna, dressing for, 64
Turkey
  ground, 33
  nutrients in, 74–75
  as Powerfood, 14
  spinach and, 39–40
Turkey bacon, uses for, 41
Turkey Lasagna, 50
Turkey sandwich, best and worst, 129
Turmeric, nutrients in, 82–83
Turnip greens, nutrients in, 78–79
Turnips, nutrients in, 86–87
TV, overeating and, 33
Twinkies, deep-fried, as worst food, 96

Vegetable juice, nutrients in, 92–93
Vegetables. *See also specific vegetables*
  color of, revealing health benefits, 34
  diet success and, 8
  length of freshness of, 60–61
  for moistening ground beef, 43
  nutrients in, 71
  as Powerfood, 11–12
  signs of freshness of, 48

sneaking into meals, 39, 44–45
  for teeth cleaning, 65
  underconsumption of, 53
Venison, nutrients in, 80–81
Vinegar
  for lowering blood glucose, 29
  for weight loss, 58
Vitamin C, exercise and, 49
Vitamins, in 100 best foods chart, 71
V8 juice, for preventing prostate cancer, 37

Walnuts, for sleep, 28
Water, for reducing hunger, 6, 68
Watercress, nutrients in, 86–87
Watermelon, nutrients in, 86–87
Weigh-ins, 172
Weight lifting, in Abs Diet, 8, 139–55
Weight loss
  high expectations for, 5
  maintaining, 172
  for medical reasons, 162–63
  promoting, with
    alcohol, 56
    calcium, 12, 71
    carbohydrate control, 37–38
    cereal, 31–32
    dairy products, 12
    diet and exercise, 2–3, 8, 158
    everyday movement, 160–61
    grapefruit, 32
    pickles, 58
    soups, 28–29
    tea, 46
    vinegar, 58
Wendy's, best and worst meals from, 119
Wheat germ, nutrients in, 76–77
Whey protein
  nutrients in, 92–93
  as Powerfood, 17
  in ricotta cheese, 50
  for smoothies, 131
Whole-grain foods
  breads, 16, 49, 68, 88–89
  cereals, 16, 90–91
  for lower weight, 13
  in 100 best foods chart, 71
Wine, best choice of, 37
Worst foods, 94–100
Wrap, spicy, best and worst, 129

Yogurt
  frozen, 39
  nutrients in, 72–73
  plain, 37
  for smoothies, 131
  as snack, 41–42
  for tooth health, 65

Zinc, for preventing overeating, 60

Also available from Rodale

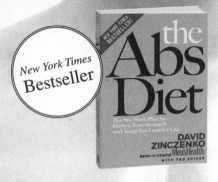

New York Times **Bestseller**

The Abs Diet, by Men's Health editor-in-chief David Zinczenko, has helped hundreds of thousands lose pounds quickly and dramatically reshape their bodies. The secret is the 12 Abs Diet Powerfoods. Now, in just 6 weeks, you too can achieve a flatter stomach and better shape—and learn how to stay lean and healthy for life.

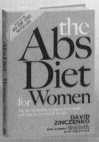

Tailored specifically to a woman's unique needs, **The Abs Diet for Women** includes an osteoporosis prevention plan, a postpartum workout for new moms, a stress-burning workout chapter, and much more.

The Abs Diet Eat Right Every Time Guide makes eating smart and healthy easy no matter where you are—at home, in the supermarket, even at the fast food counter.

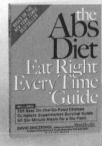

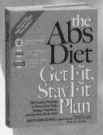

Featuring the revolutionary, 6-week, ABS3 workout plan, **The Abs Diet Get Fit, Stay Fit Plan** features hundreds of exercises and dozens of workout programs to suit every lifestyle, mood, location, and training need.

Discover 150 quick, easy, and delicious recipes in **The Abs Diet 6-Minute Meals for 6-Pack Abs**, and take control of your food choices—in less time than it takes to make it through the drive-thru.

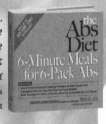

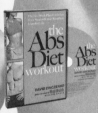

The Abs Diet Workout DVD offers the simplest, most effective plan ever developed to strip away belly fat and replace it with lean, toned, head-turning muscle in just 6 weeks.

Combining metabolism-boosting speed intervals, fat-burning resistance training, and an awesome gut-busting abs routine, **The Abs Diet Workout 2** DVD will take your body to a whole new level.

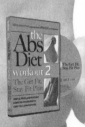

FREE 10-DAY TRIAL!

Create an interactive, personalized nutrition and fitness program, accessible 24/7 on your computer. It's sure to deliver great abs in just 6 weeks. Start today at www.AbsDiet.com/10daysfree

AVAILABLE WHEREVER BOOKS AND DVDS ARE SOLD OR VISIT ABSDIET.COM